Migraine & Head

Symptoms, causes, orthodox treatment and
how herbal medicine will help.

Other published and forthcoming titles
in the series include:

IBS & Colitis

Arthritis & Rheumatism

Anxiety & Tension

Menopause

Asthma & Bronchitis

For full details please send for a free copy of the latest catalogue.
See back cover for address.

Migraine & Headaches

Jill Wright MNIMH

HERBAL HEALTH

Published in 2002 by
How To Books Ltd, 3 Newtec Place,
Magdalen Road, Oxford OX4 1RE, United Kingdom
Tel: (01865) 793806   Fax: (01865) 248780
email: info@howtobooks.co.uk
www.howtobooks.co.uk

All rights reserved. No part of this work may be reproduced or
stored in an information retrieval system (other than for
purposes of review), without the express permission of the
publisher in writing.

© Copyright 2002 Jill Wright

British Library Cataloguing in Publication Data
A catalogue record for this book is available from
the British Library

Edited by Diana Brueton
Cover design by Shireen Nathoo Design, London
Produced for How To Books by Deer Park Productions
Designed and typeset by Shireen Nathoo Design, London
Printed and bound in Great Britain by Bell & Bain Ltd.,
Glasgow

Note: The material contained in this book is set out in good
faith for general guidance and no liability can be accepted for
loss or expense incurred as a result of relying in particular
circumstances on statements made in the book. The laws and
regulations are complex and liable to change, and readers
should check the current position with the relevant authorities
before making personal arrangements.

Herbal Health *is an imprint of*
How To Books

Contents

Preface

Do you suffer from frequent headaches and feel you need to take painkillers more often than you would like? Perhaps you find that:

- Regular use of painkillers causes side-effects.
- The headaches no longer respond to your regular painkillers.
- The headaches are interfering with work, family or social life.
- They are due to a particular emotional upset.
- They are connected with hormonal change such as PMS or menopause. The headaches may be mild or severe, cyclical or associated with seasonal change.

You may already have sought help with interpreting these symptoms, and have a diagnosis of **migraine**. If your headache is one-sided and the pain is of a throbbing nature, or if you have a tingling, cold sensation in your face and hands, visual disturbances such as flashing lights or jigsaw puzzle vision, digestive disturbance such as nausea or vomiting, and you find noise and light painful, your headache will probably be classified as a migraine.

If the pain has a burning nature and is felt in the eye as well as the head, if it comes and goes, followed by a running nose, this is known as a **cluster headache** and is another type of migraine.

If you are looking for another way of treating your

headaches, are unable to tolerate conventional medicine or find it isn't working any more, herbal medicine may offer an alternative.

I am a member of the National Institute of Medical Herbalists which was established in 1864 to maintain standards in herbal medicine. I trained for four years in herbal pharmacology, nutrition, medical sciences and herbal traditions. I offer clear, reliable advice on the safe use of herbal medicines which will help to relieve symptoms and improve your overall health. During ten years' retail and clinical practice I have answered questions every day on how to treat migraines and headaches with herbs. In this book I have set out to answer the most frequently asked questions and tell you how to find out more. Herbal medicine is the leading alternative to conventional treatment and is still the major form of medicine in many parts of the world. There are many advantages to using herbal remedies and this book will guide you simply through the process of choosing the right one. By reading this book you can:

- Discover what herbal remedies can do to relieve migraines and headaches without unpleasant side-effects.
- Learn how to combine herbs in the correct doses to achieve an individual prescription which will help your particular problems. A brief guide to how migraines and headaches develop will help you plan your own

herbal prescription as well as understand your treatments and get more out of visits to doctors and consultants.

• Find out more about food as medicine and how to maintain health by eating the right foods. A list of useful addresses and sources of information is given at the end of this book.

The advice contained in this book is for general use only. If you have an allergy, or are taking any medication or have a medical condition which may affect your use of herbal medicine, you should seek help from a qualified practitioner before using herbs at home.

Jill Wright

1

Understanding migraine and headaches

All about your head

To understand how migraines and headaches arise you need to know a little about the structure and function of organs such as blood vessels, muscles, sinuses, nerves and lymph glands in the head. This knowledge will also help you to interpret your symptoms and understand information provided by your doctors and consultants.

Blood vessels

Arteries carry blood away from the heart, veins carry blood to the heart. Both vary in size; smaller arteries are called **arterioles**, smaller veins are **venules**. Linking the two types of vessel is a huge network of tiny blood vessels called **capillaries**. It is these which provide most of the blood to our skin.

Arteries

Arteries have three layers in their walls:

- an inner surface made up of cells which are constantly being replaced as they wear out by blood cells and other components of the bloodstream.

- The middle layer consists of elastic tissue which enables the blood vessel to stretch when necessary – known as vaso-dilation – to allow the pumping movement of blood.
- The outer layer contains some muscle fibres which limit the stretch of the elastic layer so that pressure and blood flow remain even during the pumping cycle of the heart.

Blood flows from arteries to arterioles then to capillaries.

Veins

Veins are larger than arteries, they have thinner walls with more muscle and less elastic. Blood flows from capillaries to venules and finally to veins, so the pressure drops as blood flows back to the heart. Valves are found throughout the venous system and prevent blood from flowing backwards. Because there is no direct pressure from the heartbeat in the venous system, it relies on the squeezing effect of surrounding muscle movement to make blood flow.

Capillaries

Capillaries are tiny blood vessels with very thin walls, containing just a few muscle fibres. They form an immense network which would measure 60,000 miles if they were laid end to end. This makes them very important as a reservoir of blood. Their thin walls allow nutrients to pass through to surrounding tissues.

Nervous control of blood vessels

Arterioles and arteries are served by nerves which arise in the spine and carry messages using **adrenaline**. Adrenaline makes the blood vessels constrict. This type of nerve transmission is called **sympathetic**.

- Sympathetic stimulation normally increases under conditions of stress, anxiety and fear.
- Sympathetic stimulation is continuous, maintaining the blood vessels in a semi-constricted state.
- To dilate blood vessels, nerve transmission is inhibited, so that fewer messages are sent.

This puts pressure on pain receptors in blood vessel walls. It is thought that tissues next to arterioles secrete chemicals such as adenosine, histamine and lactic acid when they are short of oxygen, increasing vaso-dilation so that more blood flows to the tissues delivering oxygen. This alerts stretch receptors in the blood vessel walls and may put pressure on neighbouring tissue which causes pain.

Prostaglandins

Prostaglandins are so named because of the original site of their discovery – the prostate gland. They are made from arachidonic acid and are sometimes known as local hormones. They are secreted by body tissue and blood cells and act directly on blood vessel walls. They can act on target tissue (such as arteriole walls) directly or make tissues more responsive to other hormones. Aspirin inhibits the production of some chemicals such as prostaglandin E which mediates pain and fever. It is thought that prostaglandins causing vaso-spasm are involved in migraines and headaches.

Histamine

Histamine acts like a prostaglandin, although it is not chemically identical. It dilates arterioles and makes capillaries leaky, causing swelling.

Sinuses

Sinuses are hollow spaces in the bones of the head above the eyes (frontal) and below (maxillary). They are lined with mucous membranes which produce a starchy liquid keeping their surfaces moist. The sinuses are linked to the nose and throat passageways by narrow tubes called **ducts**. Infections pass along these ducts causing sinusitis.

Muscles of the head and neck

The face has many muscles which enable facial expression and movements of eyes and mouth. The crown of the head is covered not by muscle but by a large, wide tendon which joins with the muscle of the forehead (frontal) and the back of the head (occipital). The neck muscles – trapezius and sternocleidomastoidus – join the head at the nape of the neck. It is these which take the strain of poor posture or remaining in the same position for too long.

The muscles of the eyes may become painful if focus is maintained for too long at the same point, for example watching TV or reading. The same happens to facial muscles where squinting or frowning constantly may cause pain and spasm. Laughing too much doesn't appear to have the same painful effect!

Nerve supply to the head

The head is served by twelve different major nerves which start in the brain and serve eyes, nose, ears, mouth, face and neck. Nervous transmission occurs both towards peripheral tissue – conveying motor messages to muscles – and back to the brain, carrying sensory messages such as pain, cold, heat etc.

- The **trigeminal nerve** serves the eye, jaw, skin and mucous membranes of the head. This nerve can become inflamed by infection of the sinuses and may cause severe pain in any of these areas.
- The **vagus nerve** connects the brain to the stomach, lungs and heart. Pressure on this nerve or oxygen shortage may account for some of the digestive symptoms – such as nausea and vomiting – which accompany migraines.

- The **hypothalamus** is a group of nerve cells which regulates all autonomic (non-conscious) actions of the body, such as digestion.
- The **pituitary** is a group of nerve cells which makes stimulating factors to increase the production of hormones in other organs.

Endorphins

Endorphins are chemical messengers which mediate messages about pain. They are natural pain-relieving opiates, found in large amounts in the hypothalamus and pituitary.

Lymph glands

Lymph glands are found in the back of the neck and under the chin. You can often feel swollen ones just behind the ears when you have a cold or sore throat. Lymph glands are nodes in the **lymph channels** which contain collections of immune cells. These cells multiply when some infections occur, which is why they appear swollen and painful. Lymph channels have very thin walls and valves to prevent back-flow. They collect excess fluid from local tissues and capillaries as well as removing fats from the digestive system. The fluid is squeezed along by the action of surrounding muscles, as in the veins. When the lymph nodes at the back of the head swell, they cause pain which can spread over the whole area and cause muscular spasm.

Meninges

Meninges are membranes which line the skull and protect the brain. They secrete cerebro-spinal fluid which keeps them lubricated and provides protective insulation.

The mind

The mind is still poorly defined and understood although it is quoted so often as the major influence on many ailments. It is the store of memories, the source of analysis and humour, the controller of feelings, the generator of ideas and the mould of personality, yet no one has found the key to where these vital elements are situated or how the matrix known as our mind stays together (or falls apart).

What happens when a headache occurs

- Parts of the meninges, arteries and some nerves in the head carry special **nerve cells** which transmit pain messages when they are stretched, compressed, irritated by chemicals or deprived of oxygen.
- Muscles also contain **pain receptors** which are stimulated by chemicals secreted during over-exercise or prolonged tension. The pain which these convey is what we commonly call a headache.
- Irritation of **nerve fibres** can cause interference in vision and a burning pain known as **neuralgia** which is

a characteristic of cluster headaches and may be
associated with sinus infection.

The difference between a migraine and a headache

Headaches

Headaches are usually bi-lateral – they are felt on both
sides of the head. The pain is continuous until relieved by
medicine and often linked to common triggers such as
tiredness, excess alcohol, menstruation etc. Although they
may be severe they usually respond to over-the-counter
painkillers. It is said that **psychogenic headaches**
(possibly caused by depression) do not respond to
painkillers. They may be linked to changes in natural
endorphin levels.

Migraines

Migraines are generally one-sided and the pain is
throbbing – like a pulse. They occur with or without
known triggers and may last for several days. They do not
respond to regular painkillers. They are often preceded by
warning signs – called **auras** by some. These include
coldness and tingling around the mouth and in the
hands, flashing lights, spots or wavy lines in the vision,
which can be one-sided. These may be caused by
ischaemia – reduced blood supply due to intense vaso-
constriction – or by pressure of swollen tissue

surrounding the nerve. Some time after the initial phase of cerebral vaso-constriction – contraction of blood vessels in the brain – an intense pain begins, usually in one area, often above the eye. This pain tends to pulsate for hours or days and is thought to be due to intense extra-cerebral vaso-dilation – expansion of blood vessels outside the brain. It is frequently accompanied by sweating, nausea and vomiting. Noise and light usually make migraines much worse. General 'fuzziness' and mild pain may persist for days after the main event has subsided.

Cluster headaches

Cluster headaches are migraines which occur as a series of episodes – clusters – happening over a week or two. Pain is one-sided, and usually felt in the eye, around the eyelid and behind the nose. It has a burning character and when it ceases mucus drips from the nose. Researchers find that young men and menopausal women are more prone to this type of migraine. A common factor has not been identified.

Causes of headaches

- chemical irritation
- food intolerance
- medicines
- ischaemia and tiredness

- muscle tension and postural problems
- arthritis
- infections
- high blood pressure
- neuritis
- menopause
- tumours.

Chemical irritation

A number of chemicals can irritate pain receptors in arteries and nerves. The most common are alcohol and toxins produced by bacteria. Many industrial chemicals produce headaches if inhaled excessively.

Food intolerance

Foods containing tyramine (cheese, red wine, beef extracts, yeast extracts) cause excessive vaso-dilation in sensitive people. Foods containing methylxanthines (coffee, chocolate, tea, cola) cause constriction of cerebral blood vessels.

Medicines

Some medicines, such as the SSRI anti-depressants (the 'Prozac family') cause vaso-constriction which results in a fierce headache in the first few weeks of use. Some drugs used to control high blood pressure cause headache, probably by vaso-dilation.

Ischaemia and tiredness

Ischaemia means lack of blood. It happens when the blood vessels constrict excessively which lowers oxygen levels. This stimulates pain receptors in the artery walls. Although migraine involves vaso-dilation as well as vaso-constriction, many headaches are caused by vaso-constriction alone. Tiredness headaches are of this type. You can see this in a person's face, which is paler than usual, their hands feel cold and they feel unable to warm up.

Muscle tension and postural problems

Muscles may become over-tense when you are feeling stressed or anxious. In this state muscle fibres are stimulated by sympathetic messages from the brain. Generally the purpose of this is to prepare the body for fight or flight from danger.

Muscular stiffness and pain may also occur when the same posture is maintained for too long, for example bending over a piece of work or leaning the head back to look up. This causes pain due to vaso-constriction, ischaemia and a build-up of waste products (such as lactic acid) from muscle contraction.

Pain breeds spasm – muscles around the area contract to protect it. If this occurs in shoulder muscles (a common postural problem) pain may spread to the back of the head – a typical tension headache.

Arthritis

Pressure from worn, damaged or inflamed joints in the
neck may directly affect nerves by pressing on them. Pain
also occurs because muscles become spasmodic around
the area. Some people suffer headaches because their jaw
bones are misaligned, causing pressure on nerves and
muscular tension.

Infections

Cold and flu viruses release toxins which irritate tissues
and stimulate pain receptors. This is felt as a headache
and aching limbs. Many other febrile infections have the
same effect.

- **Meningitis**. Some bacteria and viruses can invade the
  meninges and cause irritation which causes a severe
  headache. This generally has a sudden onset,
  accompanied by rashes, fever, weakness, confusion and
  feeling very unwell. *This type of headache is not to be
  treated by herbs* – immediate treatment in hospital is
  required. If there is any doubt in your mind as to the
  cause of the headache, phone your doctor and describe
  all the symptoms, saying when they started.
- **Sinusitis**. Some infections penetrate the sinuses and
  cause inflammation with swollen tissues and increased
  mucus secretion. This causes severe burning pain in the
  forehead, under the eyes and behind the nose,
  extending to teeth on occasions.

High blood pressure

Distension of blood vessels with extremely high blood pressure causes a headache, most typically on rising in the morning. It is commonly felt in the back of the head.

Neuritis

Inflammation of the nerves can cause severe pain – called neuralgia – although it is not strictly speaking a headache. The most commonly affected nerve is the trigeminal, affecting eye, ear and jaw.

Menopause

After menopause the blood platelet cells release less mono-amine oxidase, which destroys serotonin (a cerebral vaso-constrictor). Increased circulating serotonin is also responsible for stimulation of pain receptors in the blood vessels and constriction of their walls.

Tumours

Tumours cause pain by distortion and pressure on surrounding tissues and organs. The pain is generally severe, doesn't go away and steadily gets worse. It is usually accompanied by odd sensations, deficits and disturbances which reflect damage to nerve centres in the brain. You need to seek advice from your doctor if your headache has these features.

2

What conventional medicine can offer

Conventional treatment for headaches

For general headaches a variety of painkillers – also called analgesics – are available over the counter. There are three main groups according to the main active compound:

- aspirin
- paracetamol
- codeine.

Many brand named preparations combine these elements with added caffeine. The recommended doses have been included here so that you can make useful comparisons with herbal compounds later.

Aspirin

Aspirin's chemical name is acetyl salicylic acid. It is taken in 300mg tablets, two at one time.

How it works
Aspirin is thought to inhibit the production of pain transmittors in the brain. It also reduces inflammation and fever by inhibiting the release of prostaglandins which mediate these processes.

Disadvantages
Aspirin is highly acidic and rapidly erodes the stomach
lining, causing bleeding and ulceration with over-use.
High or rapidly repeated doses also irritate the nerves
which supply the ear causing tinnitus – whistling noises –
which continue as long as aspirin is in the body.

Paracetamol

Paracetamol's chemical name is acetamenophen. It is
taken in 500mg tablets, two at one time. The
recommended maximum is four doses daily.

How it works
Paracetamol inhibits the brain's production of pain
transmittors. Unlike aspirin it is not acidic, so it does not
affect the digestion. Some people experience a lighter
mood and drowsiness when using paracetamol.

Disadvantages
In large doses paracetamol causes irreversible damage to
the liver. There is also some fear that chronic use of
paracetamol may damage the kidneys and bladder.

Codeine

Codeine is prepared as codeine phosphate. It is usually
taken in a compound remedy, 30mg to 500mg of
paracetamol for example. Dihydrocodeine is a much
stronger preparation which is also used in 30mg doses.

How it works
Codeine is a member of the opiate family. It inhibits activity of neurotransmittors in the brain and the spinal cord. This means that it affects all autonomic activities – digestion, breathing and heart rate, as well as the reception of pain messages in the brain.

Brand names
- Co-dodamol – codeine and paracetamol
- Solpadol – codeine and paracetamol
- Migraleve – codeine and paracetamol
- Veganin – aspirin, paracetamol, codeine
- Codydramol – dihydrocodeine and paracetamol
- Remedeine – dihydrocodeine and paracetamol.

Disadvantages
Codeine halts digestive movement, causing constipation, and commonly causes vomiting in sensitive individuals.

Analgesics with caffeine

Caffeine is added to analgesic preparations in small doses. For comparison a cup of fresh coffee contains 150mg caffeine.

How it works
Caffine is thought to improve the absorption of the other components, although the mechanism isn't fully understood. It dilates all blood vessels except those in the brain, which it constricts. This may explain the ischaemic pain of direct use and the rebound dilatory pain of withdrawal.

Brand names
- Anadin – aspirin and caffeine
- Anadin Extra – aspirin, paracetamol, caffeine
- Disprin Extra – aspirin and paracetamol
- Hedex Extra – paracetamol and caffeine.

Disadvantages
Caffeine increases the heart rate and causes insomnia. It causes headaches in some individuals and withdrawal may cause headaches in regular consumers.

Conventional treatment for migraines

Anti-inflammatories

These are not usually used for headaches but some migraine sufferers find them helpful.

How they work
Anti-inflammatories inhibit the production of prostaglandins which mediate inflammatory processes such as swelling and leaky capillaries. It is thought that compounds similar to the inflammatory prostaglandins are responsible for migrainous changes in blood vessels.

Brand names
- Clotam (tolfenamic acid).

Disadvantages
Frequent use can cause heartburn and damage the stomach lining.

Serotonin (5HT$_1$) agonists

Serotonin agonists are used when attacks occur.

How they work
They increase the action of serotonin – a neurotransmittor – on blood vessel walls and in the brain. This causes vaso-constriction and increases clotting. It relieves the painful vaso-dilation of migraine.

Brand names
- Sumatriptan – also known as Imigran
- Naratriptan, Rizatriptan, Zolmitriptan are new variants of this preparation.

Disadvantages
Serotonin agonists can reduce blood flow to heart muscle and raise blood pressure. They cause drowsiness at the beginning of treatment.

Ergot alkaloids (ergotamine, dihydroergotamine)

These chemicals are derived from a fungus which grows on damp rye and has a very colourful history, being blamed for visions and demonic possessions in the Middle Ages as well as giving rise to hallucogenic drugs today. They are used at the onset of a migraine attack.

How it works
Ergotamine causes immediate and intense vaso-constriction of the extra cerebral arteries.

Brand names
- Migril (ergotamine)
- Cafergot (ergotamine)
- Lingraine (ergotamine)
- Migranal (dihydroergotamine).

Disadvantages
Tissues may become deprived of oxygen because of the intensity of vaso-constriction caused by this drug. At worst necrosis (tissue death) and gangrene may occur. Ischaemia and irritation of the digestive tract, as well as disturbance of vagus nerve control can result in diarrhoea and vomiting.

Serotonin antagonists and anti-histamines

These are used prophylactically, that is to prevent attacks from happening.

How they work
They prevent the vaso-dilatory effect of histamine and the vaso-constrictory effects of serotonin.

Brand names
- Pizotifen
- Sanomigran.

Disadvantages
They cause drowsiness, dry mouth and increased appetite, promoting weight gain. They also reduce muscle responses, so can cause clumsiness.

Beta blockers

How they work
Beta blockers prevent vaso-constrictive sympathetic nerve messages from acting at receptor sites.

Disadvantages
Beta blockers prevent bronchial dilation, so can cause asthma. Tiredness and cold extremities are frequent problems, with low blood pressure and heart rate.

Anti-depressants

How they work
Some anti-depressants prevent serotonin from being destroyed. This increases vaso-constriction of cerebral blood vessels.

Brand names
- Amitriptyline
- Clomipramine
- Dothiepin
- Imipramine.

Disadvantages
Anti-depressants cause dry mouth and drowsiness if taken during the day.

Other drugs for relieving migraine

Clonidine, methysergide and sodium valproate are used mainly under hospital supervision, because of their serious side-effects. They are used for their vaso-constrictory and sedative effects.

In addition to those directly acting drugs mentioned above, doctors may prescribe contraceptive pills or HRT to effect a change in women's hormone levels. This may alleviate migraines in some women.

❧ 3 ❧

The alternative approach

When prescribing for headache and migraine a herbalist takes into account all the factors which may contribute to the development of these conditions. These include lifestyle, diet and other areas of imbalance such as digestion or the hormonal system. The herbalist then seeks herbs which treat the patient wholistically.

Using herbs to treat migraines and headaches

Herbal treatment is aimed at preventing rather than relieving pain. Herbs will be taken regularly for several months to effect a change in the pattern of blood vessel movement and achieve a better emotional balance.

Aims of herbal treatment

- prevent excessive vaso-dilation and constriction
- relieve muscular tension
- balance hormones
- improve digestion
- relieve sinus congestion
- relieve pain.

To achieve these aims we use:
- anti-migraine herbs
- circulatory tonics
- rubefacients
- relaxants
- digestive tonics
- hormonal herbs
- pain relievers
- mucous membrane tonics
- decongestants.

The patient would be prescribed circulatory tonics, which improve blood flow and ease vasco-constriction. Relaxants are used to reduce the stimulant effects of stress such as vaso-constriction. Hormonal agents can correct imbalances which may precipitate migraines, while mucous membrane tonics and decongestants relieve congestion which may cause headaches. Digestive tonics can reduce nausea and improve general energy levels which may affect the incidence of headaches and migraines.

How herbs work

Herbs contain small quantities of chemicals, compared to modern pharmaceutical products which extract or synthesise one chemical in much larger amounts. This means there is no danger of sudden physiological changes which cause side-effects. For example, valarian appears to improve the quality of your sleep as well as helping you to dose off and doesn't cause a sluggish feeling in the morning, because the chemicals it contains are in very small amounts and don't last long in the body. This lower level of activity may be disappointing if you want to be 'knocked out' but using herbs like valerian as part of a plan to restore sleep patterns can be an effective alternative to stronger, single chemicals like the well-known sedative valium (derived originally from valerian).

Most herbs contain a large number of active constituents which work together to create one or more effects. The more we find out about herbs, the more we realise that each constituent is a valued part of the whole, negative effects balanced by positive ones. A good example follows.

Recently much has been made of a research trial which showed that a St John's wort preparation made liver enzymes more active, which reduced the effect of other drugs taken at the same time because they were metabolised before reaching their target. The St John's wort preparation used was standardised to contain a larger amount of one constituent – hypercin – than all the others. Not only has hypericin failed to show anti-depressant activity on its own in repeated trials, but another ingredient – hyperforin, has been shown to counterbalance hypercin in its effect on other drugs and doctors in Germany continue to prescribe it as a favoured anti-depressant. Similar bad publicity surrounds liquorice, where glycyrrhizin is thought to raise blood pressure, but in fact dozens of other constituents act to lower it, in particular by diuresis (elimination of water).

There are many more examples of this sort of balanced action. Where two or more constituents act together to create the same effect this is known as synergy. These are particular features of herbal medicine which enable it to support the wholistic approach very well.

How long do herbs take to work?

Although some herbs act swiftly, like the relaxant valerian, herbal remedies generally act slowly and their effect is cumulative. They gently rebalance physiological processes, as though switch after switch is thrown until the full effect is achieved. This can take weeks, sometimes months, but it is worth waiting for, as the risk of side-effects is very low due to the tiny amounts of chemicals involved.

How do herbal remedies get to their target?

Herbal compounds need to be absorbed across the wall of the digestive tract, so they have to be released from their structures (stem, root, leaf, flower or berry etc) first of all. Hot water and alcohol do some of this job for us, so that teas and tinctures are more easily absorbed than tablets and capsules, which need to be broken down physically before the active chemicals are separated from the inert matter to which they are attached. All food and medicine passes through the liver (in the blood circulation) before it finally enters the body tissues, where it is used.

Sometimes chemical compounds need help in crossing through the wall of the digestive tract in the blood stream. Carrier chemicals can be attached to compounds and ferry them through channels in the gut lining. Hydrochloride is frequently found to be part of conventional drug names as it has this function.

Herbal compounds often have an advantage over synthesised chemicals in this respect, they have naturally occurring carrier chemicals already attached to them. This is what is meant by affinity. Herbs are said to have a greater affinity for the human body, like spare parts, dedicated to a particular engine made by the same manufacturer.

Are herbs safe?

All the herbs which British Herbalists use are safe when used in the correct dose for the right ailment. The herbs mentioned in this book have been selected for their safety in untrained hands, although you may need professional help with your diagnosis. The National Institute of Medical Herbalists (NIMH see page 125) maintains an extensive data band and works with government watchbodies to ensure safety of its herbs. Recently some attention was given to the group of compounds called pyrrolizidine alkaloids, present in several plants including comfrey, because they can cause (reversible) damage to the liver if ingested in large quantities. The evidence of comfrey is not based on human case studies and the research involved feeding rats exclusively on large amounts of comfrey. There is only one reported case of human toxicity world-wide, which concerned a woman who took comfrey tea many times a day concurrently with illegal drugs in high doses over a long period. Several governments, including that of Britain, made moves to ban its use. After extensive discussions with the NIMH, it was agreed to limit use to the guidelines given above, and restrict the root (which contains more PAs) to external use only. In this way herbalists acknowledge the potential risk and demonstrate the history of safe use.

Combining herbs with orthodox medication

Some drugs are altered by liver enzymes, so that they enter the main blood circulation in a different form. Some herbs (especially bitters) stimulate the liver cells to work harder, or cause more liver cells to be active and this can affect other drugs because the liver removes them from circulation before they have had a chance to do their work. Digoxin is one of these and is also a drug with 'a narrow theraputic window'. This means that the difference between an insufficient, a beneficial and a harmful dose is very small, so that small changes in the amount getting through to the bloodstream may result in the drug not working as it should. Two other drugs like this are Cyclosporin, used to prevent transplant rejection, and Phenytoin, an anti-epileptic. It is very important to check with a qualified herbalist and let your doctor know if you are adding herbal medicine to medication you are currently using.

There are many herbs which can be taken safely with other medicines, so don't feel deterred from trying, but do seek professional advice. Herbs can be used to offset the side-effects of necessary medication, like indigestion or nausea. They may enable you to take less of a remedy which you need, but which has troublesome side-effects. The important thing is how you feel, and that you don't endanger your health. It may be simple to ask your doctor to monitor blood levels of drugs and adjust the dose if necessary.

It would not be wise to embark on herbal medicine without medical supervision if you are on anti-psychotic medication, as you may not be aware that your mental condition has deteriorated when your current medication ceases to work. You may have strong feelings about the disadvantages of your drugs, but may not realise how your behaviour is changing and affecting others badly. It is possible to have herbal medicine for other complaints while on medication for psychosis, but you must consult your doctor first and allow yourself to be monitored.

If you are on chemotherapy for cancer, it would be better to wait until your treatment has finished before taking herbal medicine, unless you are looking for help with troublesome side effects such as nausea or diarrhoea. Several herbs can help here without reducing the effectiveness of your anti-cancer drugs.

Drugs to be careful with	Conditions to be careful with
Digoxin	Pregnancy
Phenytoin	Epilepsy
Anti-psychotics	Schizophrenia, psychosis
Immune suppressants	Organ transplants
Anti-cancer drugs	Allergies

Sometimes over the counter herbal medicines are labelled with contra-indications. This is required by law in Germany. It means for example that you will be told if you shouldn't take the medicine if you are pregnant, taking another specific medication, have an allergy or a certain medical condition. This will become more common in Europe in the future.

The advantages of using whole plant preparations

Herbalists insist on using whole, unaltered products to guarantee the sort of benefits we claim for them. We believe that plants would only have gained a historical reputation for certain effects if their constituents were robust enough to maintain the same effect wherever they were grown or whatever minor differences there might be between local plant populations. If only one variety in one particular year made someone feel better, its reputation would not have stood the test of time.

The current trend, based on scientific research, is to standardise the process of growing, harvesting and storing herbs, so that their use is sustainable and patients get the best value from them. Medical herbalists also recommend using whole, unaltered preparations, as nature presented them, so that each constituent is represented in its natural amounts. This is the type of preparation on which traditional knowledge is based. It is also useful to remember that patients vary much more than plants do!

The affinity of herbs

Many herbs show a greater affinity for the human body than synthetic medicines. This is because they have compounds and molecules attached which make them more easily absorbed into body cells and tissues. These are often in the sugar family. Some are known as glycosides and these and their relatives, monosaccharides, are attracting a lot of interest in the modern research world. These carrier chemicals enable herbal compounds to enter target cells more easily, and may explain how herbs can have an effect, even at quite low doses.

The constituents of herbs

Another advantage of herbal medicine is that there are so
many different plants with similar actions, but different
combinations of constituents. You can change from one to
the other to avoid becoming tolerant or developing
sensitivities. For example, there are many anti-
inflammatory herbs, each with its own supplementary
actions including hormonal, diuretic, anti-spasmodic and
relaxing effects. Herbs may act on several different aspects
of a condition at the same time, like garlic which
provides help for our circulation on several levels. As an
antibiotic it repairs the damage caused by wear and tear
on the insides of our blood vessels. As a digestive
stimulant it helps the absorption of sugars and fats from
the bloodstream. As a circulatory tonic it reduces the
stickiness of platelets, dilates the capillaries, causes mild
sweating and increases kidney activity, so it helps to
protect against strokes and lowers blood pressure slightly.

Herbal applications

Herbal remedies include conventional applications such
as:

- anti-migraine
- hormonal agents
- pain relievers
- decongestants.

There are also herbs whose actions are not found in conventional drug descriptions. Mostly this is because of their complexity which is best reflected in the older names for their applications. We can include here:

- circulatory tonics
- digestive tonics
- rubefacients
- mucous membrane tonics.

Anti-migraine herbs

There is only one herb – feverfew – which is considered a general anti-migraine herb. It has a range of actions, relieving pain, controlling prostaglandin, production and improving digestion.

Circulatory tonics

Circulatory tonics increase the flow of blood to skin and muscles by local irritation, and when taken internally they cause sweating (diaphoresis) which brings with it dilation of blood vessels in the skin. They may dilate blood vessel walls by nerve action – these are the peripheral circulatory tonics. Some circulatory tonics act on the heart to improve performance. These are called centrally acting agents and are mostly used by individuals with specific circulatory problems.

Rubefacients are applied to the skin, where they irritate nerve endings in capillaries and cause redness, which is a sign of greater blood flow through dilated vessels. This in turn causes better perfusion of joints and muscles, relieving them of metabolic wastes which may be causing pain. Very strong rubefacients, such as chilli, have a 'counter-irritant' action, that is the heat overwhelms pain receptors, so that fewer messages are received in the brain.

Aromatic essential oils are almost all rubefacient in a gentle way, so are recommended for regular use in massage for relaxing muscles and relieving pain.

Rubefacients

Rubefacients mildly irritate the skin, producing redness and warmth caused by increased blood flow to the area. This helps to eliminate by-products of metabolism which cause pain, such as lactic acid in tense muscles. The term rubefacient comes from Latin: *rube* – red, *facient* – makes.

Relaxants

Herbal relaxants relieve tension and restore nervous activity to a normal level, whereas sedatives reduce brain activity to below normal functioning level. This can improve concentration rather than impairing it, so it is a good example of a balancing action for which herbs are well known. These herbs work in two ways:

- Nervine relaxants act centrally, by reducing the brain's sensitivity to nerve messages from the periphery (skin, joints, muscles etc).

- Muscle relaxants act peripherally (on nerve centres in the spinal cord, or on nerve endings in the skin), reducing the number of messages sent from the periphery to the brain.

Many herbs have both central and peripheral actions. Relaxants provide pain relief.

Digestive tonics

Digestive tonics work by stimulating digestive secretions in the mouth, stomach, pancreas and liver. Bitters are noted for their action on the liver, increasing bile flow, which emulsifies fats and transports excess from the bloodstream. Pungent herbs (hot spices) irritate linings which respond by increased secretion of digestive enzymes. These break down starch, fat and protein as well as transporting essential vitamins and minerals across the gut wall into the blood circulation. Aromatic herbs stimulate the digestive tract in a similar way, though more gently, and they reduce bacterial fermentation which causes wind and colic. They usually also contain bitters. The aromatic bitters are well known as part of the British cookery tradition, especially in association with meat dishes.

Tonic Bitters

One of the unique aspects of herbs are the bitters. These were the mainstay of herbal manufacturers years ago. 'Tonic bitters' were sold in every pharmacy, and 'tonic

stout' was prescribed by doctors on the NHS for elderly
patients as well as breastfeeding mums until the early
1970s. Many of the famous herbal tonics are still based on
bitters, nearly every country has a national favourite. The
French drink gentian wine, Swedes export their bitters,
the British put theirs in stouts and beers, Italians prefer
vermouth, Mexicans use angostura which gave us pink
gin.

How bitters work
Bitter taste buds are located at the back of your tongue.
They are designed to detect poisons and trigger a gag
reflex, so you spit out food which is bad for you. Humans
can overcome the bitter revulsion reflex by three methods:
telling ourselves it's good for us, adding nice flavours or
adding alcohol! The body however, still working to the
primeval instruction handbook, initiates a process to rid
the body of unwanted chemicals. The liver produces more
enzymes and bile in response to messages sent in the
brain from the taste-buds. Saliva flows abundantly to
cleanse the mouth, activity in the stomach and pancreas
increases, resulting in better absorption of nutrients and
elimination of toxins. Pre-dinner drinks are good for you
after all!

A recent hospital trial showed that patients who
received nasty tasting medicine recovered more quickly
than those whose medicine tasted bland. The effect was
thought to be psychological, patients felt better because
they thought their horrible medicine was more effective.

Herbalists think that the bitter effect might have played a tonic role in this experiment.

Hormonal agents

Some herbs provide chemicals which behave like hormones in the human body; the most well known are phyto-oestrogens. These have a number of actions. Some occupy sites that human hormones might take up and so block an action, giving a protective effect against cancers which 'feed' on hormones such as oestrogen. Other herbs appear to reduce fibroid growth and excessive menstrual bleeding by an unknown hormonal action, these are often referred to as astringents by herbalists.

Some herbs contains oestrogen-like compounds which appear to relieve menopausal problems such as hot flushes and diminished bone density. We can select the right sort of hormonal herb for our wholistic purpose, for example black cohosh relieves hot flushes and protects against breast-cell overgrowth so is ideal for women who have had breast cancer, or have an increased risk factor for it. This herb also increases circulation and is mildly anti-inflammatory, so for menopausal women with arthritis it seems ideal. Some herbs, such as liquorice, act on the adrenal gland, and so help to restore the function of this organ after prolonged use of steroids.

The hormonal effects of herbs are the subject of a great deal of research which will, we hope, help to explain their traditional use in helping problems of hormone imbalance.

Pain relievers

Pain relievers are also known as analgesics and anodynes.
There are three different types of analgesic.

- Central acting analgesics stop the brain from receiving
  messages from the periphery. Passionflower, lettuce leaf,
  poppy and St John's wort work in this way.
- Herbs such as silver birch and wintergreen have a local
  action and are applied topically.
- Anti-inflammatories, like the ones described above, and
  muscle relaxants such as cramp bark and wild yam, act
  on the processes which cause pain. Herbal pain relief is
  a little slower than conventional medicine, it can
  sometimes take two to three days for a full effect to
  build up, but it's well worth waiting for as it seems to
  last longer and there are no associated problems.

Mucous membrane tonics

Mucous membrane tonics reduce over-secretion of mucus,
swelling and inflammation in the linings of the airways
and sinuses. The action on membranes is also referred to
as astringent drawing tissues together. Some of these herbs
increase the flow of thinner secretions which 'washes out'
thickened, infected mucus. Mucous membrane tonics are
often called anti-catarrhals. Their main effects are on the
airways of the head.

Decongestants

Decongestants work by stimulating the linings of the nose and sinuses to produce thinner secretions, (eucalyptus, peppermint), or by reducing the number of bacteria causing thickened mucus (eucalyptus), or by constricting the small blood vessels which cause swelling of the membranes (ephedra).

Wholistic therapies

Herbs can help you manage or overcome migraines but you should also consider other therapeutic ideas to maintain improvement. A herbalist prescribing in consultation would make recommendations for exercises and other therapies based on your individual life-style and general health status.

Yoga

Yoga is a system of exercises developed over thousands of years in India. It includes methods for meditation which are extremely useful to relax the mind and breathing exercises which help to regulate oxygen levels. Postural exercises relax and tone the muscles as well as improving joint condition and posture. These are all aspects of relaxation which is essential to defeating migraine.

You can find an evening or daytime yoga class in every local education authority programme, as it is very popular and well accepted in Britain today.

Massage

There are many different types of massage, including foot massage. It can have a very beneficial effect on migraine. It is noted for lowering blood pressure and pulse rate, albeit temporarily, and should be deeply relaxing. Massage therapies are the main focus of most complementary therapy clinics. You can also take evening classes in massage if you want to extend your knowledge and improve your techniques.

Exercise

It is very important to make opportunities for regular daily exercise as this improves circulation and helps to reduce muscular tension. Walking is ideal, and greatly underrated as a form of exercise. Over-use of cars has deprived many people of a daily walk to school, shops or work, which they struggle to replace with an hour's energetic exercise once a week in a gym. Park and stride would be a good maxim!

Gardening is a very relaxing, energetic form of exercise. Forget the low maintenance, one foot in the gravel approach. Go for soul-soothing flowers and digging and plenty of it! You might even produce a few organic vegetables and herbs while you're at it.

4

Directory of useful herbs

You will need to use a number of strategies to relieve migraines and headaches. Dietary approaches are covered in Chapter 6 on nutrition. You can use the information in this section to select the right herbs. The case histories in Chapter 7 guide you in building classic recipes or tailoring one to your own individual needs.

Herbs are usually categorised by their actions, and each herb will have some primary and some secondary actions. In some the actions are of equal importance. To treat headache and migraine we use anti-migraine herbs, circulatory tonics, rubefacients, relaxants, digestive tonics, hormonal herbs, pain relievers, mucous membrane tonics and decongestants. When you read the case histories later, you will see how this directory can be used to pick herbs from the various categories to suit your individual needs.

ANTI MIGRAINE HERBS

Feverfew

There is really only one herb in this category, whose actions span
the circulatory, relaxant and pain-relieving groups. Its traditional
use for migraine is well known and its effectiveness well
documented.

Feverfew

Latin name	Tanacetum parthenium
Origin	Europe
Part used	Leaf
Dose	1 teaspoon per cup
	Tincture 4ml, 1-3 times daily
Constituents	Volatile oil (pinene, angelate, farnesine),
	bitter sesquiterpines, pyrethrin, tannins
Primary actions	Pain relieving
	Anti-inflammatory
Secondary actions	Relieves fever
	Digestive tonic
How it works	The sesquiterpenes inhibit production of
	prostaglandins, which mediate inflammation
	and swelling in arteries. They are also mildly
	anti-spasmodic and reduce serotonin
	secretion from blood platelets, which
	prevents its potent vaso-constrictory activity.
	Many people find the volatile oils mildly
	relaxing, the angelate component may be
	responsible for this effect.

Caution   A very few people find that feverfew makes
                       their mouth sore. This effect is overcome by
                       using tablets with plenty of water or putting
                       the tincture in a drink.

CIRCULATORY TONICS

Buckwheat	Horsechestnut	Rue
Gingko	Motherwort	
Hawthorn	Passionflower	

Note – if you are suffering from hot flushes and night sweats,
you will find the spicy circulatory tonics, (ginger, chilli, mustard,
horseradish) can make your symptoms worse, so to deal with
circulatory problems you will need herbs which are not
diaphoretic (sweat – inducing).

Buckwheat

(see Chapter 6)

Ginkgo

Latin name	Ginkgo biloba
Origin	Asia
Part used	Leaf
Dose	1 teaspoon per cup
	Tincture 4ml, 3 times daily
Constituents	Ginkgolides, flavonoids
Primary action	Circulatory tonic
Secondary action	Anti-inflammatory
How it works	Research on ginkgo is growing, but little is

known of its main chemical constituents. The ginkgolides stop blood cells called platelets from sticking together, so this provides the anti-thrombotic effect. Platelet aggregation occurs in allergic reactions, so ginkgo is also used in asthma and hayfever. Flavonoids are also noted for their stabilising effect on blood vessel walls, so this might be another reason why ginkgo inhibits inflammation (where water escapes from the leaky blood vessels and causes swelling). Its main reputation, newly arrived in Europe from the far East, is for improving circulation to the brain. Modern research has confirmed this effect. The flavonoids and ginkgolides probably act together to dilate and repair blood vessels, so help to protect against strokes. One study showed that it only had these effects in elderly people and showed no effect in younger men and women!

Growing guide	Suitable for parks and estates only, as it is a very tall tree. Very tolerant of modern pollution.
Caution	Not to be used with anti-coagulant medication such as warfarin and heparin.

Hawthorn

Latin name	Crataegus oxyacanthoides
Origin	Europe
Part used	Fruits

Dose	1 teaspoon per cup
	Tincture 2ml, 3 times daily
Constituents	Alkaloids, flavonoids, cyanogenic glycosides, saponins, tannins, phenols
Primary action	Heart tonic
Secondary actions	Anti-spasmodic
	Diuretic
How it works	The flavonoids and glycosides improve the heart muscle's ability to use oxygen and reduce the fragility of small blood vessels. They are anti-spasmodic and mildly relaxing, so they dilate the blood vessels a little, which lowers blood pressure, and they help to stabilise the heart rate. The saponins are mildly anti-coagulant so reduce the tendency to thrombosis. When taken fresh the berries contain vitamin C, which aids the repair of blood vessel walls and keeps them smooth, so hindering plaque and damage from cholesterol deposits. Used as a gargle, the phenols and tannins are useful for sore throats. One of the alkaloids, amygdalin, is now called laetrile and has a new reputation as an anti-cancer agent. The flowers have some of the actions of the berries and can also be made into a tea.
Growing guide	Will tolerate impossible conditions! Wild, wet and windy landscapes as well as urban streets. A very undervalued tree.
Caution	Not to be taken with anti-clotting medication

such as warfarin, heparin, etc or anti-arythmic drugs such as digoxin.

Horsechestnut

Latin name	Aesculus hippocastanum
Origin	Europe, Asia
Part used	Fruit, bark
Dose	1 teaspoon per cup
	Tincture 4ml, 1-3 times daily
Constituents	Saponins, tannins, glycosides, coumarins, tiglic, angelic acid, flavones
Primary actions	Venous tonic
	Astringent
Secondary actions	Diuretic
	Anti-inflammatory
How it works	The flavonoids and glycosides are deposited in the blood vessel walls, so improve their strength and elasticity. They are diuretic, so the extra elimination of water contributes to the reduction in swelling (oedema) which often accompanies weak, bulging (varicose) veins. The coumarins and saponins reduce clotting, so protect against thrombosis. The glycosides and flavones also inhibit the inflammatory process, so help to relieve phlebitis. Applied topically, tannins also reduce bacterial infection as well as inflammation so are useful to treat leg ulcers. The acids are probably febrifuge (reduce temperature) as well as being mildly relaxant.

	This may account for the traditional use of horsechestnut in fevers.
Growing guide	Only suitable for estate and park gardening, easy to germinate.
Caution	Not to be taken with anti-coagulant medication such as warfarin, heparin etc.

Motherwort

(see hormonal herbs)

Prickly Ash

Latin name	Zanthoxylum Americaum
Origin	America
Part used	Berries
Dose	$^1/2$ teaspoon per cup, 1-2 cups per day
	Tincture 2ml, 1-2 times daily
Constituents	Resin, volatile oil, bitters, coumarins, alkaloids, tannin
Primary actions	Circulatory stimulant
	Increases sweating
Secondary actions	Tonic
	Anti-spasmodic
How it works	It is not yet known which compounds cause the effects on peripheral circulation. Coumarins relax muscles in the gut and relieve spasm. Bitters increase liver and digestive secretions. Volatile oil and resins create warmth when applied to the skin, so may also be responsible for the internal circulatory effect. It is also known as

toothache weed in some parts of America,
which confirms that it has been used as a
pain reliever as well.

Rue

Latin name	Ruta graveolens
Origin	Europe
Part used	Leaf
Dose	1/2 teaspoon per cup
	Tincture 2ml, 1-3 times daily
Constituents	Volatile oil, flavonoids, coumarins, alkaloids, acids, phenols
Primary action	Anti-inflammatory
Secondary action	Anti-spasmodic
How it works	The volatile oil contains anti-spasmodic and antiseptic compounds, which help to relax and repair blood vessel walls. The flavonoids also relax blood vessels and reduce their leakiness which inhibits inflammation. Coumarins are anti-coagulant, so help to protect against thrombosis. The main action of the alkaloids isn't known, they may be responsible for its reputation in relieving palpitations. When the herb is applied topically it reduces pain; this action is probably due to the volatile oil. Rue has a long tradition of use for migraines in Europe.
Growing guide	From seed under glass, needs full sun.
Caution	Some people are highly allergic to this plant, and develop severe blistering on contact.

They are very few, but you should try a small skin patch test with your remedy first. Not to be taken with anti-coagulant medication such as warfarin, heparin, etc.

RUBEFACIENT ESSENTIAL OILS

Cedarwood	Pine	Wintergreen
Juniper	Rosemary	
Lavender	Thyme	

These are all used topically (in massage or bath) and contain mildly irritating constituents which increase blood flow to the skin. This in turn causes increased perfusion of tissues underneath, reversing vaso-constriction and relaxing muscles.

RELAXANTS

Chamomile	Lemon balm	Valerian
Cramp bark	Limeflowers	Vervein
Kava-kava	Skullcap	

Chamomile

Latin name   Matricaria recutita (this plant has been renamed several times recently, so you must specify small, cone-headed flowers with single row of petals. This is currently called German chamomile)

Origin   Europe

Part used	Flowers
Dose	1 teaspoon per cup, 1-3 cups per day
	Tincture 5ml, 1-3 times daily
Constituents	Volatile oil, flavonoids, coumarins, valerianic acid, sesquiterpene bitters, salicylates, tannins
Primary action	Relaxant
Secondary action	Digestive tonic
How it works	Chamomile is one of the most complex herbs in common use. It has a little of almost every action shown by plants.The volatile oil acts on the brain to reduce sensitivity as well as being mildly antiseptic and anti-inflammatory when applied topically. Flavonoids are mildly diuretic, coumarins relax visceral muscle by acting on local nerve centres. The volatile oil is carminative (reduces bacterial ferment and wind in the gut).Sesquiterpene bitters stimulate bile production in the liver and there are bitter glycosides which add to this action. Anti-inflammatory salicylates are present in small quantities. Tannins astringe and tone the wall of the gut, alleviating diarrhoea.
Growing guide	Annual. Sow seeds each year in pots, window boxes or scatter freely in a sunny position in spring.

Cramp Bark

Latin name	Viburnum opulus
Origin	Europe

Part used	Bark
Dose	1 teaspoon per cup 1-3 cups per day
	Tincture 3ml, 1-3 times daily
Constituents	Viburnine, tannin, valerianic acid, coumarins
Primary action	Anti-spasmodic
Secondary actions	Relaxant
	Digestive tonic
How it works	Coumarins and other constituents relax muscle by reducing the number of messages sent to the brain. They affect both digestive muscle and skeletal muscle. Valerianic acid acts on the brain to reduce reception of messages, producing a feeling of relaxation. Viburnine is bitter, so has a tonic effect on digestion. The tannins reduce the free flow of water through the gut wall, so help to alleviate diarrhoea.
Growing guide	Easy to grow shrub, green-white flower heads in early spring, available in most garden centres as snowball bush.
Caution	Some people feel drowsy when they take this herb, so wait one hour after drinking for the first time to see what effect it has on you before driving or operating machinery.

Kava-kava

Latin name	Piper methysticum
Origin	South Sea Islands
Part used	Root
Dose	1 teaspoon per cup, 1-2 cups per day

	Tincture 3ml, 1-2 times daily
Constituents	Pyrones, piperidine alkaloids, glycosides, mucilage
Primary actions	Relaxant
	Anti-depressant
Secondary actions	Anti-spasmodic
	Diuretic
How it works	Not much is known about the actions of kava-kava, though research is increasing as it becomes popular. The pyrones and piperidines act centrally (on the brain) to reduce sensitivity to pain. Applied topically it is rubefacient and numbing. It also has a reputation for relieving fatigue, so in some books it is referred to as a stimulant. It is best to view it like alcohol, relaxing and stimulating at the same time, with some effects of intoxication at high doses.
Growing guide	It has not been tried in the British Isles.

Lemon balm

Latin name	Melissa officinalis
Origin	Europe
Part used	Leaf
Dose	1 teaspoon per cup 1-3 cups per day
	Tincture 4ml, 1-3 times daily
Constituents	Volatile oil, flavonoids, phenols, triterpenes, tannins
Primary actions	Relaxant
	Digestive tonic

Secondary actions	Anti-viral
	Anti-thyroid
How it works	The volatile oil has a central relaxing effect (on the brain) as well as reducing thyroid hormone stimulation of other systems. It also inhibits the growth of viruses such as herpes by giving a sort of repellant protection to the tissues, and possibly penetrating viral coating. The phenols add to this effect and help to dispel bacteria in the gut. Triterpenes are bitter, so stimulate digestive secretions, and tannins astringe the wall of the gut, alleviating diarrhoea.
Growing guide	You will rarely have to resort to seed, nearly everyone has some lemon balm to give away. It seeds itself like mad, tolerates any soil and will grow in pots.

Limeflowers

Latin name	Tilia europaea
Origin	Europe
Part used	Leaf and flower
Dose	1 teaspoon per cup, 1-2 cups per day
	Tincture 4ml, 1-3 times daily
Constituents	Volatile oil, flavonoids, phenols, mucilage, tannins
Primary actions	Relaxant
	Lowers blood pressure
Secondary actions	Increases sweating
	Anti-spasmodic

How it works	The volatile oil reduces the brain's sensitivity to pain messages, mucilage soothes the stomach and gut wall and flavonoids make blood vessels less fragile. Phenols are antiseptic and diaphoretic (increase sweating), which induces dilation of blood vessels. The overall effect is to calm and lower blood pressure. Limeflowers is a particularly nice tasting tea.
Growing guide	Too large a tree for the average garden, a most magnificent specimen can be seen at Kew Gardens in London.

Skullcap

Latin name	Scutellaria laterifolia
Origin	America
Part used	Leaf
Dose	1 teaspoon per cup, 1-2 cups per day
	Tincture 3ml, 1-3 times daily
Constituents	Flavonoids, glycosides, iridoids, volatile oil, tannin
Primary actions	Relaxant
Secondary actions	Anti-spasmodic
	Possibly anti-inflammatory
How it works	Little is known about the active constituents of American skullcap as most research is based on a Chinese variant. We rely on the tradition of use for our knowledge of its actions. The anti-inflammatory effect is present in the Chinese variety and it is very

likely that both varieties have the same constituents. American Skullcap is noted for its central (brain) calming effect, flavonoids stabilise blood vessel walls and contribute to its mooted anti-inflammatory effect, as well as mildly increasing the elimination of water via the kidneys. It has a long traditional use for neurological diseases such as epilepsy and motor neurone diseases.

Growing guide Prefers damp soil. Sow under glass and plant out in early summer in a warm, damp spot (pond-side, bog-garden).

Valerian

Latin name	Valeriana officinalis
Origin	Europe
Part used	Root
Dose	1 teaspoon per cup, one cup per night Tincture 2-5ml, nightly
Constituents	Valerianic acid, alkaloids, glycosides, tannins, choline, flavonoids, valepotriates, iridoids
Primary actions	Relaxant/sedative
Secondary actions	Anti-spasmodic
How it works	Valerianic acid and valepotriates reduce excitability of the brain and feelings of anxiety. Best used at night as it is on the borderline between relaxants and sedatives. Flavonoids are mildly diuretic (increase water elimination).
Growing guide	Sow directly in a sunny spot with damp soil in early spring.

Vervein

Latin name	Verbena officinalis
Origin	Europe
Part used	Leaf, flower
Dose	1 teaspoon per cup, 1-3 cups per day
	Tincture 3ml, 1-3 times daily
Constituents	Glycosides, iridoids, bitters, volatile oil, alkaloids, mucilage
Primary actions	Relaxant
	Bitter digestive tonic
Secondary actions	Anti-depressant
	Anti-viral
How it works	Not all actions are clearly understood. Bitters stimulate liver and digestive secretions, unknown constituents act on the brain to reduce sensitivity to pain and increase feelings of well-being. These are probably found in the volatile oil, which is responsible for the anti-viral effect, acting as a repellant in the tissues of the body. This is known as the 'constitutional effect' which French aromatherapists call the *terrain theory*. The whole herb has some pain relieving action when applied as a poultice to inflamed joints and muscles.
Growing guide	Sow under glass, plant out in late spring. Vervein is a very delicate looking plant which will seed itself readily in sunny spots.

DIGESTIVE TONICS

Pungent digestive tonics	Aromatic digestive tonics
Chilli	Lemon balm
Galangal	Rosemary
Ginger	Sage
Horseradish	Thyme

Chilli, ginger and horseradish

All these may be taken freely in foods.

Galangal

Latin name	Alpinia officinarum
Origin	Asia
Part used	Rhizome
Dose	1/2 teaspoon per cup, 1-2 cups per day Tincture 3ml, 1-3 times daily. Also used in cooking, especially Indonesian dishes. Tastes of cloves and ginger.
Constituents	Volatile oil, sesquiterpenes, probably acetoxyeugenol
Primary action	Digestive tonic
Secondary action	Carminative
How it works	The aromatic and pungent elements of the volatile oil stimulate digestive secretions and the bitter sesquiterpenes increase liver activity. Some varieties contain acetoxyeugenol, which is antiseptic and carminative (dispels wind and colic). It is likely that commercial stocks of galangal

contain different varieties.

Growing guide   Not grown in Britain.

Lemon Balm

(see Relaxants)

Rosemary

Latin name	Rosemarinus officinalis
Origin	Europe
Part used	Leaf (oil externally)
Dose	1 teaspoon per cup, 1-2 cups per day
	Tincture 3ml, 1-3 times daily
Constituents	Volatile oil, phenols, flavonoids, tannins,
	bitters, resin
Primary actions	Digestive tonic
	Circulatory tonic
Secondary action	Anti-inflammatory
How it works	The volatile oil contains several compounds

The volatile oil contains several compounds which stimulate nerve endings and produce a sense of warmth. They also stimulate the lining of the digestive system, which responds by secreting more digestive juices. The bitters stimulate the liver to produce more bile, so that fatty meat and nut dishes are more easily digested, hence the famous combination of rosemary and lamb. The phenols are mildly antiseptic, they reduce fermentation in the gut, alleviating wind and colic. The volatile oil components do penetrate brain tissue, where they facilitate nerve message transmission. This action has given rise to the traditional view that rosemary improves memory. Research trials using oils of sage and rosemary with elderly residents of nursing homes have shown reliably to improve mental function.

Sage (see hormonal balancers)

Latin name	Salvia officianalis
Origin	Europe
Part used	Leaf
Constituents	Volatile oil, phenols, flavonoids, tannins, bitters, resin
Primary actions	Digestive tonic
	Circulatory tonic
Secondary action	Hormonal
How it works	As rosemary (above), although not associated with memory function. Sage is often combined with pork.
Growing guide	From cuttings in a sunny spot.

Thyme

Latin name	Thymus vulgaris
Origin	Europe
Part used	Leaf
Constituents	Volatile oil, phenols, flavonoids, tannins, bitters, resin
Primary actions	Antibacterial
	Digestive tonic
Secondary action	Anti-inflammatory

| *How it works* | As rosemary (above). The same volatile oil gives an antibacterial and anti-inflammatory effect, especially in the lungs, hence its traditional use in asthma. |
| *Growing guide* | Easily grown from cuttings in light soil. |

HORMONAL HERBS

Anemone	Hops	Sage
Black cohosh	Motherwort	White deadnettle
Chasteberry	Red clover	Wild yam

Anemone

Latin name	Anemone pulsatilla
Origin	Europe, Asia
Part used	Leaf and flower
Dose	$1/4$ teaspoon to 1 cup
	Tincture 1ml, 3 times daily
Constituent	Volatile oil, saponins, tannins, resin, camphor
Primary actions	Relaxant nervine
	Anti-spasmodic
Secondary actions	Hormonal agent
	Alterative
How it works	Saponins are often related in structure to hormones. In anemone they are stimulant to the liver, increasing bile flow and so helping to improve metabolism of nutrients, especially fats. This action may help to protect against the development of

gallstones, and the hormonal saponins affect both male and female hormone structure, though the mechanism is not understood. The volatile oil and tannins may be responsible for the alterative action – this is an old term used to describe herbs which relieve both viral and bacterial infections. The nearest modern equivalent is an antibiotic, but antibiotics only act on bacteria, whereas the herbal compounds appear to increase the body's resistance to a variety of organisms. It was once considered a specific cure for measles. Its main use today is for nervous exhaustion, pain and inflammation in the reproductive system, especially in menopause. It is observed to stimulate secretion of all mucous membranes, and this may account for its use as a remedy for vaginal dryness.

Growing guide   From bulbs in a well drained, sunny spot.
Caution   The fresh plant should not be used as the oil is irritating to skin and mucous membranes.

Black cohosh

Latin name   Cimicifuga racemosa
Origin   North America
Part used   Rhizome
Dose   1/2 teaspoon per cup
    Tincture 2ml, 2-3 times daily
Constituents   Glycosides, bitters, isoflavones, volatile oil, tannins

Primary action	Hormonal agent
Secondary actions	Anti-spasmodic
	Anti-inflammatory
	Circulatory tonic
How it works	Black cohosh has another American Indian name, 'squaw vine', which suggests its traditional use in female complaints. Its isoflavones bind to oestrogen receptors in the body, so have some oestrogenic effects, and the same chemicals are anti-spasmodic, helping to relax blood vessels, lower blood pressure and slow pulse rate. These actions also reduce the severity of palpitations. Its bitters help to remove sugars and fats from the bloodstream, which adds to the circulatory tonic effect. Some research has shown that black cohosh has been used successfully in conjunction with drug treatment for breast cancer. It appeared to reduce the severity of hot flushes and reduce the proliferation of breast tissue. This is what herbalists call a balancing action but it is not not fully understood. It is very likely that other so-called oestrogenic herbs will have the same anti-cancer effects, but more research into how they interact with drugs is needed before we can recommend them for use during chemotherapy. To be on the safe side, we recommend using herbs after chemotherapy is finished as drugs like

tamoxifen still offer the best outcomes for breast cancer sufferers.

Growing guide	Tolerates semi-shade and prefers damp soil. Used to be a popular Victorian garden plant. Tall white spires of flowers, 4ft high perennial.

Chasteberry

Latin name	Vitex Agnus castus
Origin	Europe, Asia
Part used	Seed
Dose	1/2 teaspoon per cup
	Tincture 2ml, 1-2 times daily
Constituents	Volatile oil, alkaloids, bitters
Primary action	Hormonal balancer
Secondary actions	Anti-spasmodic
	Diuretic
How it works	The 'chaste' aspects of the herb refer to its effects on men, where it has a noted sexual sedative quality. Its other name was monk's pepper! Its volatile oil acts on the pituitary gland and its connections with the hypothalamus, increasing dopamine effects in that area. It also increases the activity of luteinising hormone, so increases both progesterone and oestrogen production in the ovary, and it is noted for reducing excessive prolactin. This is what accounts for the hormone balancing effect, and its traditional use for PMT symptoms, such as

breast tenderness and bloating. The diuretic effect is probably also due to the volatile oil, and contributes to the relief of water retention and bloating. The bitters stimulate digestion, improving fat metabolism and nutrient absorption.

Hops

Latin name	Humulus lupulus
Origin	Europe
Part used	Strobiles (flowers)
Dose	1 teaspoon to 1 cup
	Tincture 2ml, 3 times daily
Constituents	Volatile oil, bitter resin, tannins, valerianic acid, oestrogenic compounds, flavonoids
Primary actions	Sedative
	Hormonal agent
Secondary actions	Bitter digestive
	Diuretic
How it works	Hops is very bitter, which helps to preserve beer by inhibiting bacteria. The same action reduces fermentation and wind in the gut. The bitter-tasting compounds stimulate the production of bile in the liver. This action helps to prevent and relieve gallstones. The flavonoids are diuretic (promote the elimination of water) so they relieve water retention and the same group of chemicals contains oestrogenic substances which help to regulate periods. It is a useful relaxant

nervine for irritability and for women who are at risk of developing gallstones. It is also possible that moderate, quality beer-drinking may be of benefit to menopausal women!

Growing guide   Very easy from layered cuttings, prefers sun and is a rampant climber

Motherwort

Latin name	Leonurus cardiaca
Origin	Europe
Part used	Leaf and flower
Dose	1 teaspoon to 1cup
	Tincture 4ml, 3 times daily
Constituents	Alkaloids, bitter glycosides, flavonoids, caffeic acid, volatile oil
Primary actions	Sedative nervine
	Relaxing circulatory tonic
Secondary actions	Anti-spasmodic
	Uterine tonic
How it works	Motherwort offers an example of synergistic actions. The alkaloids, glycosides and flavonoids work together to reduce smooth (internal) muscle spasm, including the muscles of the heart, as its Latin name suggests. The alkaloids have a relaxing effect on the brain, so a feeling of calm results. Together these actions relieve heart palpitations and nervous tension in menopause. Motherwort's name gives away its traditional use as a uterine tonic. 'Mother'

is the old name for womb. It prepares the
womb for easier contractions during labour
and helps to reduce fibroid proliferation. It is
not known which chemicals are responsible
for these actions, but the general effect makes
us assign it to the progesteronic group when
mixing herbs for balance.

Growing guide   Tolerates most soils, prefers chalk, seeds itself
in gardens.

Red Clover

Latin name	Trofolium pratense
Origin	Europe
Part used	Flowers
Dose	1 teaspoon per cup
	Tincture 4ml, 3 times daily
Constituents	Flavonoids, isoflavones, phenolic and
	cyanogenic glycosides, coumarins
Primary actions	Depurative
	Hormonal agent
Secondary actions	Anti-spasmodic
	Diuretic
	Anti-thrombotic circulatory tonic
How it works	The flavonoids are diuretic, so help the
	kidneys eliminate water and soluble toxins.
	This may account for red clover's traditional
	use as a depurative in skin conditions. The
	phenols are antibiotic, so add to the
	cleansing effect on the skin. Coumarins
	reduce the stickiness of blood cells called

platelets, which helps to prevent clots forming and causing thrombosis. Isoflavones are now known to be responsible for the hormonal action as they mimic oestrogen and provide precursors for oestrogen production. This explains the use of red clover tea to relieve hot flushes. Its oestrogenic effects contribute to heart and bone health in menopause. Cyanogenic glycosides and coumarins are also anti-spasmodic as they relax smooth muscle, which can lower blood pressure a little by allowing blood vessels to dilate.

Growing guide   Easy from seed, rather invasive, prefers sun.
Caution   Not to be taken with other anti-clotting medication, such as warfarin and heparin.

Sage

Latin name	Salvia officinalis
Origin	Europe
Part used	Leaf
Dose	1 teaspoon per cup
	Tincture 4ml, 3 times daily
Constituents	Volatile oil, flavonoids, phenols, tannins, oestrogenic, saponins
Primary actions	Antiseptic, antibiotic
	Astringent
	Hormonal agent
Secondary actions	Digestive stimulant
	Anti-spasmodic
	Relaxant

How it works   The tannins and phenols act together to
subdue bacteria on direct contact in the
mouth and throat and when used as a wash
for infected skin. The phenols also act in the
gut to reduce bacterial fermentation so they
relieve wind. It is likely that the antibiotic
phenols are responsible for sage's reputation
for relieving night sweats in tuberculosis and
glandular fever. The bitters stimulate
digestion of nutrients, especially fats, hence
its use with rich meat and nut dishes. The
hormonal compounds relieve hot flushes as
well as night sweats, and reduce milk
secretion, so help when weaning infants.
New research into the essential oils has
confirmed its mildly relaxing qualities and
shown its ability to improve mental function
in the elderly. This is a supreme herb for
women in menopause, as it relieves hot
flushes and indigestion, relaxes and improves
the mind!

Growing guide   Very tolerant of soils, prefers sunny spot, easy
from seed under glass.

White deadnettle

Latin name   Lamium album
Origin   Europe
Part used   Leaf
Dose   1 teaspoon per cup
Tincture 4ml, 3 times daily

Constituents	Tannins, polypeptides (amines), flavonoids, alkaloids, saponins, mucilage
Primary actions	Astringent
	Uterine tonic
Secondary actions	Anti-spasmodic
	Prostate remedy
How it works	The polypeptides are probably responsible for this herb's ability to check heavy bleeding in menstruation and when applied to wounds topically. The saponins are likely to be hormonal and account for the anti-spasmodic and co-ordinating effects on uterine (womb) muscle. This is another herb to use in combination for women with heavy menstrual bleeding or fibroids.
Growing guide	From seed sown directly in spring.

Wild Yam

Latin name	Dioscorea villosa
Origin	South America
Part used	Rhizome
Dose	1 teaspoon per cup
	Tincture 4ml, 3 times daily
Constituents	Steroidal saponins, alkaloids, tannins, phytosterols
Primary actions	Anti-spasmodic
	Hormonal agent
Secondary actions	Digestive tonic
	Anti-inflammatory
How it works	It isn't known which constituents provide the

anti-spasmodic action. For many years this was considered to be its main action, relieving colic and constipation. When modern research revealed the hormonal action of the saponins and other phytosterols, wild yam became a favoured remedy for oestrogen deficiency in menopause. It also has a strong reputation for relieving arthritic stiffness and pain. This action may be due to the phytosterols (plant hormones). This plant was used to synthesise oestradiol when the contraceptive pill was first manufactured.

Growing guide   Not tried in Britain, poly tunnels might enable it to grow.

PAIN RELIEVERS

See Relaxants and Anti-inflammatories.

MUCOUS MEMBRANE TONICS

Elderflower	Ground Ivy	Ribwort
Eyebright		

Elderflower

Latin name	Euphrasia officinalis
Origin	Europe
Part used	Leaf

Dose	1 teaspoon per cup
	Tincture 4ml, 1-3 times daily
Constituents	Volatile oil, flavonoids, tannins, phenols, mucilage, ursolic acid, sterols, linolenic acid
Primary actions	Anti-catarrhal
	Expectorant
Secondary actions	Anti-inflammatory
	Diaphoretic
How it works	Elderflower usually forms a part of remedies for colds, because it offers something for every aspect of this complaint. The flavonoids and tannins reduce inflammation and bacterial growth. The mucilage soothes and the phenols are also antibacterial. The volatile oil contains several components which cause diaphoresis – dilation of skin capillaries and sweating. This lowers temperature. Elderflower's constituents reduce congestion in the sinuses but the exact mode of action cannot be explained.
Growing guide	Elderflower is a very attractive small tree, with clusters of black berries in the autumn which birds and wine-makers love. Grow from cuttings and be patient, the bark of an old elder is very beautiful.

Eyebright

Latin name	Euphrasia officinalis
Origin	Europe
Part used	Leaf

Dose	1 teaspoon per cup
	Tincture 4ml, 1-3 times daily
Constituents	Glycosides (including aucubin), volatile oil, tannins, alkaloids, phenols, choline
Primary actions	Anti-catarrhal
	Astringent
Secondary actions	Anti-inflammatory
	Anti-bacterial
How it works	Phenols and tannins are antibacterial. Eyebright is commonly used as an eye-wash, where the tannins act directly on bacterial and viral conjunctivitis. Its constituents are thought to act synergistically to reduce pain and congestion in nose, sinuses and middle ear. Its astringent action reduces swelling and over-secretion.
Growing guide	Eyebright prefers chalky soil but will tolerate rich soil. Grow from seed sown directly in spring.

Ground ivy

Latin name	Glechoma hederacea
Origin	Europe
Part used	Leaf
Dose	1 teaspoon per cup
	Tincture 4ml, 1-3 times daily
Constituents	Tannins, volatile oil, choline, saponins, flavonoids, bitters
Primary actions	Anti-catarrhal
	Expectorant

Secondary action	Digestive tonic
How it works	Bitters stimulate digestion, flavonoids stabilise capillary membranes and so are anti-inflammatory. Tannins are antibacterial where applied directly (gargle, digestive tea). Ground ivy has a long tradition of use in nervous headaches and sinusitis, for which the aromatic volatile oil is probably responsible.
Growing guide	Grow from seed sown directly in spring or under glass.

Ribwort

Latin name	Plantago lanceolata
Origin	Europe
Part used	Leaf
Dose	1 teaspoon per cup
	Tincture 4ml, 1-3 times daily
Constituents	Mucilage, glycosides, tannins
Primary actions	Anti-catarrhal
	Astringent
Secondary actions	Antiseptic
	Soothing
How it works	Ribwort's mucilage soothes the throat, its tannins are astringent, reducing bacteria on contact. The constituents work together to relieve over-secretion of mucus and swelling in the sinuses, although the exact mechanism of action is not known.
Growing Guide	This is a surprisingly elegant little plant with

black seed heads and long, glossy green
leaves. Grow from seed direct or under glass,
transplanting in spring.

DECONGESTANTS

Ephedra	Eucalyptus	Peppermint

These are primarily inhalant herbs not taken internally,
including eucalyptus and peppermint. They act by mildly
stimulating the nasal lining which causes a freer flow of mucus,
thus relieving congestion. A few herbs, such as ephedra, are
available on prescription but not over the counter.

❧ 5 ❧

Growing and making
your own herbal remedies

You can prepare herbs in a wide variety of ways to bring relief from headaches and migraines.

Types of herbal preparation

Oral remedies

Oral remedies are swallowed in measured doses. They include:

- teas
- tinctures
- syrups
- pills.

Topical remedies

Topical remedies are applied to the skin and include:

- creams
- oils
- baths
- plasters and poultices.

Oral remedies

Teas or tisanes

Teas also called tisanes can be made directly from dried herbs.

- Leaves and flowers require five minutes steeping in freshly boiled water. Always place a saucer or cover on the cup to keep in valuable aromatic ingredients. This is known as an **infusion**.
- Roots, barks, seeds and berries need boiling for five minutes in a covered pan. This is called a **decoction**.

The usual dose is one rounded teaspoon per cup (about 4g to 165ml). Regular use means one or two cups per day for several weeks. Infusions and decoctions can be drunk cold, and any flavouring can be added after steeping or boiling.

- To make an infusion steep cut leaf or flower for 5-10 minutes in boiling water.
- To make a decoction, boil cut root or bark for 5-10 minutes on the stove.

Many people ask if the dosage of dried herbs should be different from fresh herbs. As the loss of chemicals in drying may balance the greater concentration due to loss of water, it is best to simply use the same amounts whether fresh or dry. Some herbs such as lemon balm, chamomile and basil taste better when fresh and are slightly more effective but most herbs keep their medicinal qualities very well if dried carefully. Roots and barks often improve their taste with drying as they lose their acrid components and become sweeter.

Measurements

1ml = 1g
1 teaspoon = 5ml
1cup = 165ml

Tinctures are usually 1: 5, or one part herb to five parts alcoholic liquid.

Doses for adults

Adults will usually require one to three cups a day of herbal teas (whether infused or decocted), using one teaspoon of herb per cup.

Adult doses of tincture vary according to the herbs used in them. Usually half a teaspoon of single herb tinctures, three times daily is required. With great care, you can get 80 drops onto a 5ml teaspoon, so you can work out your dose that way too, and use the formula given below to calculate a child's dose. The amount of alcohol in one teaspoon of tincture is very small but you can add the remedy to hot water and allow some of the alcohol to evaporate if you wish. Elderly people may require different doses, as body weight falls, or if digestion isn't as good. One should start with a lower dose and work up if required.

Doses for children

Children require smaller doses. There are some formulae which can be used, based on a child's age. For example, divide the child's age by twenty, to give the proportion of an adult dose, i.e. 6 (years) divided by 20 = 3/10 adult dose. You also have to take into account the child's body weight, giving less if a child is underweight for his/her age.

Common doses for teas are: a tablespoon of tea to a child under 5, half a cup for a child from 5 to 10 years and a full cup from 11 years onwards. Beatrice Potter seems to agree, as Peter Rabbit was given a large spoonful of chamomile tea after he had over-eaten in Mr McGregor's garden!

Making your own formula

You can combine herbs in tincture or tea form to obtain a mixture of effects which will suit your individual needs. Start by choosing the actions that you want – for example relaxant, pain relieving, hormonal, and look for herbs which provide them. It is best to include no more than three or four herbs in one mixture, and with careful selection you can choose herbs with more than one action to match your requirements.

If you are using dried or fresh herbs to make teas, you should choose herbs which require the same sort of preparation (remember that roots, barks and seeds need boiling, leaves and flowers need infusing). You will only need one teaspoon of your mix because herbs act synergistically as you have learnt already.

Tinctures

These have become very popular in Britain, both among herbalists and consumers. They are made by soaking herbal material, finely chopped, in an alcoholic liquid about 70% proof. This could be brandy or vodka. Generally, you use one part herb to five parts liquid, so 100g to 500ml. Chop the herbs as finely as possible and cover with the alcohol. Turn, shake or stir every day for ten days. This is to ensure that every particle of herb is in contact with alcohol, otherwise moulds may develop. After ten days, strain and squeeze out the remaining 'marc' through a clean piece of material. Keep the tincture you have made in a dry bottle with a tight stopper.

This can be used in place of herbal tea. Each teaspoon of tincture generally gives the effect of a small cup of tea. Sometimes herbal constituents are extracted better by alcohol, so it is a useful way of preserving herbs. In the past, wines and vinegars were used, their trace is found in the nursery rhyme Jack and Jill where Old Dame Dob did mend Jack's nob with vinegar and brown paper.

It is obvious that these are much bigger doses than is often suggested on over-the-counter tincture bottles, where the manufacturer is more concerned with keeping the price and profit margin at an attractive level. Tinctures are more expensive than teas, and you should expect to pay between £3 and £5 for a week's supply.

Tincture of lemon balm
100g lemon balm
500ml vodka or brandy

Chop herbs finely, cover with alcohol, shake or stir daily for ten days, strain and bottle.

Herbal syrups

Herbs can be preserved in syrup but they are quite difficult to make, as the proportion of sugar to herbal material is crucial. They frequently go mouldy, however carefully you measure. There are two methods, the first is the simplest, but only keeps for a few days.

Syrup recipe 1
Place chopped herb and sugar in 1cm layers in a clean, dry jar, finishing with a sugar layer. Leave for one day. You will find a syrup has formed. You can shake the jar gently once a day until all the sugar has turned into syrup. This may take three days but you can use the product immediately.

Syrup recipe 2
Soak 4g of herb, finely chopped, in 56ml water for 12 hours. Strain and squeeze out the herbs. There should be about 45ml liquid. Add 90g sugar, stir over heat until dissolved, boil briefly, strain through a filter paper or cloth. You should have about 100ml syrup. This must be

kept in a well stoppered bottle in a cool, dry, dark cupboard. The dose would usually be 1 teaspoon at a time for children, and a dessertspoon from 11 years onwards.

Pills

These come in two main varieties: pills and capsules. In both cases, powdered herbs are used. Capsules are usually made of gelatine, although vegetarian ones can be obtained. Most are of a standard size, containing about 2g of herb. You can buy herbs ready powdered and fill your own capsules by hand. It's a very sneezy, time consuming business! Tablets are made by pressing powdered herbs into the required shape. You will need to add ingredients to make the dough stick together and the tablets hold their shape. Manufacturers usually use vegetable gums, but quite satisfactory tablets can be made at home using honey and arrowroot as binders. Pills can either be pinched off and rolled between the fingers or tablets cut by hand from dough rolled with a pin.

Buckwheat pills

2 tablespoons buckwheat flour
1 tablespoon arrowroot powder
4 teaspoons runny honey

Knead all ingredients together. Add more honey if required to achieve a malleable paste. Dust board with arrowroot, roll out, cut to shape, dry on paper overnight.

Topical remedies

There are several forms in which herbs can be applied to the outside of your body. This is known as topical application. You need to remember a little bit about skin to understand how herbs reach their target when used in this way.

The skin

Skin has several layers designed to keep water in (you suffer dehydration quickly if large areas of skin are broken) but allow moisture out when required to cool the body down by evaporation. It is covered with a cornified layer (dead cells) and wax. Blood vessels are very close to the surface, and they dilate when we are hot to allow heat out by convection. They also dilate when we are emotionally stressed, so we flush with anger, embarassment or affection. These blood vessels can constrict to conserve heat, and sometimes when we are very angry or upset we become paler than our usual colour.

Fat underneath the skin keeps heat in by insulation and protects some areas from pressure (famously the bum!). Muscle is found underneath linings below the fatty layer. If you want to reach muscles, your topical applications must somehow get through the wax, cornified layer, fat and muscle linings first. Oily preparations do penetrate through these layers to some extent.

One way of increasing penetration is to soak the skin in water for a while. This can be done in the bath, in a steam room, or on small areas with a poultice or plaster. Belladonna plasters for back pain could still be bought in the chemist's until a few years ago. Most people have heard of anti-smoking and hormone patches. These use the same principle. Back to Old Dame Dob and her vinegar on brown paper!

Four ways of increasing absorption through the skin:

- bath
- steam
- poultice
- plaster.

Creams

Creams are more complicated to make. It would be easier to choose a favourite bland cream over the counter and add aromatic oils or tinctures as you wish. If you want to try a cream, try the following recipe.

Rosemary cream
8 parts oil
1 part beeswax
a few drops essential oil

Gently heat oil and beeswax together in a bowl, set in a pan of water. When wax has melted, add essential oil and pour into pots immediately.

Greasy ointments like this are generally not considered to be good for skin conditions such as eczema, where they inhibit healing and trap heat, but they are suitable for applying as muscle and joint rubs. Their advantage over liquid preparations is that they don't drip on the floor. A cream such as the one described above could be used to make a vapour rub to help sinus-related headaches.

Massage oils

This option is useful if you want to use herbs from your garden. Simply pick a handful of fresh herbs, chop finely and cover loosely with any oil – almond, olive or even sunflower oil. Place the bowl of oil and herbs in a pan of water and put the lid on. Heat until simmering and leave on the lowest possible heat for 1-2 hours. A slow-pot can give ideal conditions for making infused oils as it maintains a constant, very low simmering temperature. Spices can also be infused in vegetable oils.

There are many essential oils available now which save you the time involved in infusing plants in oil. The easiest way to apply these is in a carrier oil such as olive, almond or coconut. A few drops to a tablespoon will suffice. You can add a dash of chilli or ginger! Massaging increases blood flow to muscles and breaks down the tension in them.

Baths

Essential oils can be added to the bath. Use a teaspoon of

unscented bubble bath or a tablespoon of milk to act as a dispersant. Relaxing bath salts are based on the same principle and available commercially, although they don't smell as nice as genuine essential oils. The relaxing effect is limited, but a helpful contribution, especially at night before bed, and there are no side-effects.

Plasters and poultices

These are used to apply steady heat or continued absorption of pain relieving or relaxing constituents to joints or muscles.

Plasters are made by melting one part of beeswax and two parts of vegetable oil, adding tincture or essential oil at the last minute. Soak a suitably sized cloth in the mix and spread out on a tray to cool and firm up. Apply to the body and cover in plastic or cling film (or paper!) and tie on with a bandage or some tight garment. The most common use is application to chest, back, abdomen and forehead. You could add a hot water bottle or hot towel wrap for extra comfort.

Poultices are similar to plasters, but consist of a 1cm thick layer of fresh or macerated herbs applied to the skin and covered with a piece of material. This was the earlier form of a plaster, but can still be immediate and effective.

Steam inhalations

Nowadays it is easy to buy good quality essential oils so it is simple to make a steam inhalant mix using a large china mug. Some chemists sell a special inhaler cup, made of plastic, which fits over the nose and mouth. You can also use the older method of covering the head with a towel and leaning over a bowl of steaming water, but this is very tedious and time-consuming. You can heat your inhalant mix in an aromatherapy oil burner, using a votive candle and adding your oil to water. This gives a gentle decongestant and relaxing effect in your room.

Dried herbs can be used for steam inhalation but they are not as strong or convenient.To be effective, you need to steam twice daily. If you are using a steam inhaler cup, you must allow the water to cool a little before allowing a child to use it, to avoid scalding if spilt.

Caution. You must never leave a naked flame unattended in a room with children and you must remember to place your burner on a heat-proof surface.

Vapour rubs

You can apply decongestant, antibacterial and relaxing herbs to your skin, by adding essential oil to a cream base and rubbing into the chest or under the nose. This is a useful method for children.

Caution. You must check that the preparation isn't too strong as most decongestants are also 'rubefacient' – they heat up the skin and may cause a burning sensation. Peppermint is especially noted for this.

Recipe for vapour rubs
5 drops essential oil in 30mg of (preferably unscented)
cream, stirred well.
Suitable oils for headache relief:
- peppermint
- eucalyptus
- chamomile (very expensive)
- rose (very, very expensive!)
- lavender.

Choosing, growing, and storing herbs

Identifying herbs in the wild

It is important first of all to know that you have the right
plant. Some botanical families include poisonous and
edible plants which look very similar and can only be
distinguished from each other by fine botanical detail,
like hemlock and valerian which have subtle differences in
stem and flower colouring. You could buy a field botany
guide, as identification of plants is a great hobby, but it
would be wiser not to select your remedies from the wild
if you are a complete beginner.

Fortunately many of the most important medicinal
herbs are garden favourites such as thyme, sage, rosemary,
lemon balm and peppermint. Most people recognise them
and they are pretty unmistakeable. Even where there are
different varieties such as the thymes and mints, they have
the same aroma and characteristics. It is better to choose

the original sort for medicinal purposes rather than a variety because it may be a more reliable source of the chemicals that you need for your remedy.

Choosing herbs

There is a system of naming plants which gives each one two Latin names – the family name comes first and has a capital letter, the individual name comes second written in lower case. The meaning is reversed in Latin, for example *Thymus vulgaris* means common thyme. This is the one you would use for cough medicine – other types, such as *Thymus aureus* (golden thyme) or *Thymus serpillus* (creeping thyme) will do no harm, but they don't have as much aroma – in fact they put most of their energy into looking pretty! The same can be said for the many lovely varieties of achillea – a cottage garden flower related to Yarrow (Achillea officinalis) The word *officinalis* in a plant's name means it was known to be used medicinally in the seventeenth century or before. You will need to specify both names when you are buying seeds or plants from nurseries. Addresses of reliable firms are given on page 124.

Growing herbs

Many of the herbs mentioned in this book can be grown in British gardens, some can be grown in pots or window ledges. Growing herbs is a very relaxing and rewarding hobby. Although most aromatic herbs originate in the

warm Mediterranean countries, they will do fine in a
sunny spot in any garden soil, even on London clay. They
do prefer well drained (slightly dry) soil, so adding grit
and compost will help them along.

If you are growing from seed, you will need to start
them off in pots first on a window ledge or in a
greenhouse. To sow seeds really successfully, you should
buy John Innes compost number 1. This contains lots of
sand and fine grit, so that water runs through quickly and
the seed doesn't sit in its own tiny puddle of water, which
causes a fungal growth gardeners call damping off.

When you have a small stem with two leaves, pull it up
gently and plant in a pot with John Innes number 2
compost. This has more soil, so that fine roots can spread
and take in water – it also contains a little more nutrient
to feed the growing plant. When your plant is about 10
cm tall or has a few branches, it's time to plant it in a
sunny spot or container, using John Innes number 3. John
Innes is a type of compost, not a brand name, so you can
ask for it at any garden nursery.

Planting out

Locate your herbs in the south west corner of your garden
if possible. Herbs don't need feeding or watering once
they have extended their roots into the garden soil (after
about a week) but containers will need to be watered as
they dry out continually. You can even grow herbs in
hanging baskets. You can use multi-purpose compost, but

you run a much greater risk of damping-off and losing seed before they even grow, which can mean a whole growing year lost. If your plants don't succeed in one spot in your garden, move them! Just dig up enough soil around the plant to ensure minimum root disturbance and put them in somewhere else. Experiment to see what works. There are plenty of herbs to choose from, so find one that suits your garden or space.

- choose a sunny spot
- add grit to improve drainage
- start tender plants under glass
- water pots and baskets daily
- move plants if they aren't happy.

Choosing the right part of the plant

It is important to know which part of the plant you need if you are going to make your own herbal remedies. Flowers, leaves, roots, bark and berries are commonly used but sometimes one part of a plant is edible whereas another part is poisonous. We eat the tuberous root of the potato but avoid the berries and we eat rhubarb stems but not the leaves. Comfrey root stores too many alkaloids which can damage the liver, whereas they are barely present in the leaf. It is common to find stems in with leaves in herbs sold over the counter, as it is difficult to separate them when preparing herbs on a large scale. If you are preparing your own you should take the trouble to rub the leaves off the stems as your remedy will be stronger without this inert woody matter.

Harvesting herbs

Choosing the right time to harvest is also important, it helps you to get the best quality of herbs in terms of the chemical constituents.

- Leaves are picked just before flowers develop.
- Flowers are picked as they come out.
- Berries as they become fully ripe, while they are still smooth and shiny.
- Bark and stem is stripped in the late spring from new branches.
- Roots are dug up in early autumn before the first frosts. Pick on a dry day, and scrub roots immediately after digging.

Storing herbs

Most plants can be used fresh, but it is more convenient to dry them for use all the year round. The rules for drying herbs are:

- as cool, fast, dark and dry as possible, with as much air circulating around the individual herbs as can be allowed.

The best way for home preservation is to hang up small bunches of herbs, loosely tied, in a dark room or shed. A washing-line strung across the attic is ideal. Hanging up in the kitchen will cause most of the colour and aroma to be lost before they dry.

Large roots should be chopped before drying, as they will prove too tough for the knife otherwise. They can be spread out in a single layer on newspapers. The newspapers should be changed when they feel very damp.

Herbal material is ready to store when it is cracking dry. This is a matter of experience. Usually leaves will simply not leave their stems until they are thoroughly dry. Roots should snap briskly or fail to bend under pressure. Berries usually give a little under thumb pressure. They are slow to dry – moulds develop if there is too much moisture so gentle heat (airing cupboard level) is helpful.

When thoroughly dry herbs should be stored in cool, dark, dry, airless conditions because sunlight destroys colour, air removes flavour and water causes moulds. Tin boxes are ideal, however plastic tubs and glass jars are OK provided they are kept in a cupboard.

- Hang leaves on branches upside down.
- Spread roots out in a single layer.
- Dry as fast as possible in cool, dark, airy place.
- Ready when cracking dry.
- Keep in cool, dark, dry, airless conditions.

~ 6 ~

Using nutrition to prevent headaches and migraines

There are many ways in which you can use diet to improve your resistance to stress, tiredness and infections, which are common causes of headaches. In this chapter you can also find out about the most common trigger foods and how they initiate migraines.

Understanding the basic principles of nutrition will help you to plan your week's eating and incorporate beneficial foods into your diet.

Achieving a balanced diet

The main aim of a healthy diet is to satisfy the need for energy, growth, repair and elimination.

Therapeutic diets

A therapeutic diet is one that addresses the needs of people with a particular complaint, for example gluten-free diets for coeliac disease, sugar-free diets for diabetes and so on.

People who suffer from headaches and migraines

should aim at a general healthy diet with special attention to the following aims;

• High vitamin and mineral content for immune defences
• Decreased saturated fats and increased essential fats for healthy mucous membranes

Daily nutritional requirements

In Britain research into food was started during World War II and was continued by the Ministry of Agriculture and Fisheries with help from the Medical Research Council. They produced guidelines on what people need to eat to keep them healthy and prevent deficiencies. These are called the minimum daily requirements and they cover the main nutrients needed by the human body. In America USDA (the United States Department of Agriculture) funds a similar programme, and its books are widely used in Britain.

Nutrition for general health

It is a mistake to look at single nutrients as being a cure for specific conditions, as almost all body processes require a broad range of nutrients to keep them running smoothly. All human cells need sugar as a fuel to perform their vital functions. Muscles use sugar for fuel as well as calcium and potassium to contract and relax. Salt (sodium) plays an essential role in getting calcium into muscle fibre cells and potassium is vital to maintain the correct amount of salt in the body. All these processes are dependent on each other and on a balanced state of nutrients in the body. This is the state of health which the herbalist tries to restore with herbal medicines and wholistic dietary advice. It is usual to divide food up into seven different categories and we should aim to eat something in each category every day.

You could use these categories to design a food diary or plan your eating for a week.

- **Protein** – cheese, meat, beans, nuts, fish
- **Starch** – bread, potatoes, pasta, roots, rice, grains
- **Vitamin A** – green, orange and yellow vegetables
- **Vitamin B** – meat, wholegrains
- **Vitamin C** – fresh fruit and green vegetables
- **Vitamin D** – fish oil and sunlight
- **Vitamin E** – wholegrains and seeds
- **Vitamin P** – also known as bioflavonoids – fresh fruit and vegetables
- **Minerals** – calcium, potassium, sodium, magnesium, zinc, phosphorus, found in vegetable and animal foods
- **Trace elements** – cobalt, copper etc , found in vegetable and animal foods
- **Fibre** – indigestible parts of vegetables and grains
- **Fat** – butter, vegetable and nut oils, margarine.

Daily requirements for nutrients

These vary according to age and occupation (whether you have an active or sedentary job). Here, we have taken the figures for sedentary workers. You can use these tables to understand information given on labelling of supplements.

- 1mg = one thousandth of 1g, 1μg = 1 millionth of 1g

	Men 35-64	Women 18-54
kcals	2,400	2,150
protein	60g	54g
calcium	500mg	500mg
iron	10mg	12mg
vitamin A	750μg	750μg
thiamin (vitamin B$_1$)	1mg	.8mg
riboflavin (vitamin B$_2$)	1.6mg	1.3mg
niacin (vitamin B)	18mg	15mg
vitamin C	30mg	30mg
vitamin D	10μg if no sunlight available	10μg if no sunlight available

Women's needs vary to a greater extent than men's because of changes taking place during pregnancy, breastfeeding, the monthly menstrual cycle and menopause. British guidelines suggest that women over 55 take fewer calories (1,900kcals) and less iron (10mg) daily. The lower iron intake is suggested because there will be no monthly losses due to menstruation and the smaller calorie intake reflects metabolic changes after the menopause.

American researchers give us figures for some of the other vital nutrients which apply to both men and women

vitamin k	70-140µg
biotin (vitamin B)	100-200µg
pantothenin (vitamin B)	4-7mg
potassium	1,875-562 mg
phosphorus	700-800mg
sodium	1,100-3,300
chloride	1,700-5,100

Canadian guidelines complete the picture, with daily requirements for men and women between 25 and 49 and recommendations for the over 50s (blank means no change).

	Men	(over 50)	women	(over 50)
vitamin E	9mg	7mg	6mg	
folacin (vitamin B)	220µg		175µg	190µg
pyridoxine (vitamin B_{12})	2µg		2µg	
magnesium	250mg		200mg	210mg
calcium	800mg		700mg	800mg
iodine	160µg		160µg	
zinc	9mg		8mg	

It is interesting to note that Canadian researchers think we need a lot more daily calcium than their British counterparts. This is because they recommend a much higher protein intake which causes greater loss of calcium from the body. You may need to take this into account when you are looking at labels on vitamin and mineral supplements.

Other minerals considered essential for daily nutrition are chromium, selenium, molybdenum, copper, manganese and fluoride. The intakes for these are generally very small figures – from .2 to .5µg. These are called trace elements.

The guidelines presented above are based on the amounts needed to stop you developing deficiency conditions, such as scurvy which develops when you don't get enough vitamin C. Some nutritionists think you need more than these if you have certain diseases, but this is a very undefined area, with lots of claims motivated by the desire to sell products. General health is achieved by eating a balance of all necessary nutrients, which will help the body grow, repair itself and resist infection.

Especially useful nutrients

Bioflavonoids

This group of chemicals includes rutin, quercitin, lutein and hesperidin. Bioflavonoids regulate the elasticity and strength of blood vessel walls. This means they will be more able to withstand changes caused by stress and illness. They are usually found accompanying vitamin C in plants, which is the reason some people say that natural vitamin C is better for you than the synthetic form. Fresh fruit will usually supply daily requirements. Some other foods also contain useful amounts of bioflavonoids.

Vitamin C, chemical name ascorbic acid

Vitamin C is involved in all energy and repair processes in the body, as well as disease resistance. It is not stored in the body, so you must take some every day.
Recommended intake of vitamin C is 30mg in Britain, 60mg in America. British figures are, as explained before, based on the amounts needed to prevent deficiency diseases. American and Canadian figures are higher because of the higher protein intake.

Vitamin C content of foods	% of daily requirement	
1 cup orange juice	124mg	200%
½ canteloupe melon	113mg	188%
1 cup broccoli cooked	98mg	163%
1 green pepper	95mg	158%
1 orange	70mg	116%
1 cup cauliflower, cooked	69mg	115%
1 cup parsley	54mg	90%
raw cabbage	33mg	55%
baked potato	26mg	43%

You should cut the vegetables just before using and cook them conservatively – that is using just enough water to cover, boil the kettle first and add to vegetables. Boil until just tender, use the water in gravy. This method conserves the vitamin C, which is lost to heat, air and water. Steaming vegetables is even better, but you will need to add salt at the table. Frozen vegetables retain some of their vitamin content, supermarket vegetables may have lost some vitamins in transport. The best vitamin content is obtained by growing your own and picking just before eating.

Essential fatty acids (EFAs)

There are two essential fatty acids, linolenic and linoleic. These are components of fats which are mainly found in plants but found in very small quantities in meat. Wild meat, also known as game, contains far more EFAs than domestic animal meat. They are needed to make cell membranes, especially in surfaces which are constantly being worn away and replaced, such as digestive tract linings. The human body cannot make these fatty acids and cell membranes cannot be made from any other type of fats. They are part of the group known as polyunsaturated fats, which includes arachidonic acid (made in the body from linoleic acid) and eicosapentoic acid (from fish). This fish oil has beneficial effects on blood circulation but is not used directly to make cell membranes. It is possible that a deficiency in these essential fatty acids (also known as omega 3 and omega 6 acids) may contribute to inflammation of the digestive tract linings, as they might be unable to secrete protective mucus efficiently.

There are few established recommendations for EFAs. American dietary researchers recommend 6g of EFAs daily, from mixed sources. British authorities suggest between 2-10g daily.

EFA content of foods, g per 100g		
	Linoleic	Linolenic
safflower oil	75g	.5g
wholemeal flour	59.4g	4.1g
barley	57.4g	6.1g
potatoes	56.5g	17.2g
green peppers	56.3g	12g
corn oil	50g	1.6g
soya beans	52g	7.4g
sunflower oil	52g	.3g
grouse	31.9g	30.3g
rabbit	20.9g	9.9g
chicken	13.5g	.7g
rapeseed oil	15.5g	10.5g

There are no figures available for hemp, evening primrose and borage oils which are reported to have higher linolenic acid levels than other oils, and are much vaunted as dietary supplements for all types of diseases. Rapeseed oil is also known as vegetable oil, it appears low in the list for linoleic acid but has the highest content of linolenic acid of all the common cooking oils. Linolenic acid is also present in useful quantities in green leaves and beans. It appears from this table that eating a mixed diet with plenty of vegetables, especially beans and greens will supply an adequate amount of both essential fatty acids without needing supplementation.

To maintain a healthy digestive system it may suffice to add 5-10ml of vegetable oils as a salad dressing to a green salad and reduce your animal fat consumption by taking low fat milk, game or white meat (or no meat), reducing cheese consumption and choosing 'white' cheeses such as Wensleydale, Caerphilly, Stilton, Lancashire, Cheshire and goats' cheeses as these contain a lot less fat than other varieties.

How to increase EFA's in your diet without increasing calories

- eat salad every day with dressing (lemon and oil)
- eat potatoes and roots instead of pasta
- cook with vegetable oils, use gentle heat for frying
- use soft vegetable margarine instead of butter
- make cakes with vegetable oils instead of hard margarine
- eat beans in salads, soups and with meals
- eat five portions of vegetables and fruit daily.

In addition, dieticians from the American Heart Association recommend that fat should only represent 30% of your calorie intake. Several books show elaborate schemes of 'calorie exchange' which are quite difficult to follow. By weight fat gives far more calories than starch, so a simpler approach might be to think in terms of a tablespoon (15ml) of fat a day from all sources. This would mean thinking carefully about cakes and pastries, which contain 'hidden fat'. The average pasty contains 50g of fat in the pastry alone! Baking fat is hydrogenated, which converts polyunsaturated fats into saturated fats. These cannot be used for cell membrane building, and leave you no room for further fat intake from healthier sources.

Foods containing bioflavonoids

Buckwheat is very rich in a bioflavonoid called rutin which helps to regulate the elasticity of blood vessels and reduce inflammatory swelling. This can help to reduce the severity of migraines. In medieval Germany rue was possibly used for the same purpose. Buckwheat is pleasant eaten as a vegetable in pancakes and stews. Buckwheat tablets are available in many health food shops.

Foods which can trigger migraines and headaches

Tyramine

Tyramine mediates the release of nor-adrenaline – a vaso-constrictory agent which can cause migraines and raise blood pressure. It is inactivated by an enzyme called monoamine oxydase (MAO). Blood platelets release less

MAO after menopause, so some women suffer more migraines then. Some antidepressants prevent MAO from destroying tyramine, so they are to be avoided by migraine sufferers along with the foods which contain it. Tyramine is contained in:

- cheese
- yeast
- beef
- beef and yeast extracts (Bovril, Marmite, Oxo)
- pickled herrings
- red wine.

Methylxanthines

Methylxanthines, including theophylline and caffeine, constrict cerebral blood vessels and dilate extra-cerebral vessels. This is why foods and drinks containing them can trigger migraines. Coffee is noted for increasing the pain of headaches, whereas tea contains other relaxant ingredients such as theobromine which balances theophyllene to some extent. Methylxanthines are found in:

- coffee
- tea
- cocoa and chocolate
- cola.

Nicotine

Nicotine is a potent vaso-constrictor. Smoking is never to be recommended, but should be especially avoided by those who are prone to headaches.

Does wheat cause headaches?

There isn't any reliable evidence that wheat causes headaches. Some researchers think that 'leaky gut syndrome' allows large proteins through into the bloodstream, where they cause a variety of reactions. The anecdotal evidence is very clouded and rarely tested.

Yeast

It doesn't seem that yeast in baked bread causes a migraine problem but further research into the effects of grains and yeasts in the human body would be very helpful.

7

Case studies

Case 1 Migraine and acid indigestion

Mr H, a 48 year old headmaster, had developed chest
pains and was burping constantly. He was no longer able
to enjoy a glass of wine and took a great number of
antacid tablets daily. He passed loose bowel motions
frequently and had poor circulation, with moderately
high blood pressure and chilblains in the winter. He said
his digestion had been poor since leaving university. He
also endured migraine attacks at least once a month, with
tingling fingers, flaming lights and vomiting. Mr H
suffered from insomnia, waking three or four times
nightly. He confessed to not enjoying sport and his only
exercise was walking the family dog in the evening. Mr H's
priority was to relieve his indigestion. His remedy was
chosen carefully to reduce muscular tension (evident in
the headaches, blood pressure and indigestion), relieve
circulatory problems and improve digestion.

The remedy

- Cramp bark – muscle relaxant.
- Chamomile – digestive tonic.
- Feverfew – migraine reliever.
- Liquorice – antacid digestive emollient.

Mr H was also prescribed slippery elm tablets and meadowsweet tea. This combination was very successful. Mr H was completely symptom-free after ten days. He continued to take medicine for three months, in which time he had one migraine. He then reduced his remedies to meadowsweet tea with 1 teaspoon daily of feverfew tincture. This continued to protect him from indigestion and migraine.

Case 2 Psychogenic headaches and fainting fits

Mrs K was a 60 year-old widow who lived alone and had been suffering from headaches for some years. The pain was located in the crown of her head and was continuous. She also reported several fainting episodes, which caused her to fall downstairs. Hospital scans had revealed nothing to account for these symptoms. She had been mugged a year previously, and following the attack, she suffered acute back pain with a degree of paralysis in her legs, had given up work and walked with a stick. She also experienced pains in her chest as well as breathlessness on climbing stairs. Her blood pressure was low and she had swollen ankles for which she was prescribed a diuretic by her doctor. Mrs K wasn't sure which area of her health she wanted help with first, so we prioritised her headaches and circulation. The remedy was aimed at relieving nervous tension which seemed to be at the root of her headaches.

The remedy

- Cramp bark – muscle relaxant.
- Hawthorn – heart tonic.
- St John's wort – relaxant, antidepressant.
- Valerian – relaxant.

Mrs K was also prescribed dandelion root and chicory coffee as a digestive tonic.

This relieved the headaches completely and Mrs K had no more fainting fits. She continued to suffer back pain and leg problems, so she was recommended osteopathic investigation and treatment.

Case 3 Muscle strain and headaches

Mr S, a 35 year-old taxi-driver with a young family, had suffered one-sided headaches once or twice monthly for five years. They started when he gave up his polytechnic studies to join the family firm. After lifting some heavy luggage into the cab boot his back muscles on one side went into spasm, requiring a visit to the local hospital casualty department. After that incident he had continued to suffer muscular pain on the same side as well as tingling in his arms and legs and a clammy feeling in his skin. He had suffered from hayfever since his early years but had no other health problems. He ate a balanced diet, supplemented by a cod-liver oil capsule, but drank very little during the day, 'an occasional cola' was all he could record.

Mr S had tried various treatments, having teeth removed, braces fitted, physiotherapy, osteopathy, yoga and massage. All of them helped a little but none were curative.

It seemed likely that Mr S was experiencing migraines with a number of causes. Driving all day, using his left arm for gear changes and lifting luggage, were creating excessive muscular tension and strain on one side of his body. Recurrent congestion due to hayfever (and earlier nasal polyps) contributed to head pain. Emotional tension as Mr S settled into his new working life probably added to the general level of tension which he acknowledged. His osteopath confirmed that the muscles on one side of his body were hypertrophic and hypertonic (larger and more tense).

The remedy

- Cramp bark – muscle relaxant.
- Valerian – relaxant.
- Elderflower – mucous membrane tonic.
- Eyebright – mucous membrane tonic.

This worked slowly. Hayfever symptoms disappeared in three weeks, muscular pains and headaches eased after two months. Mr S started a system of postural re-training called Alexander Technique which increased the improvement and he tried to remember to get out of his cab and stretch between fares.

Case 4   Hormone problems and migraines

Miss K, a 36 year-old interior designer, began to experience occasional migraine and headaches – three or four per year after the birth of her son eight years previously. She described severe pain, which didn't respond to painkillers and tingling in her hands. Since her early 20s she had noticed spots and boils on her back and chest, with more oily skin and increasing hair on her face. All these symptoms improved during pregnancy but returned afterwards. Miss K also said that she was permanently tired and her blood pressure was rather low. She ate a well-balanced diet, drank lots of water but cheese and milk products formed a large part of her protein intake.

After discussing her case history we agreed that her headaches were likely to be the result of tiredness and a hormone imbalance as well as poor circulation.

The remedy
- Chasteberry – hormonal agent.
- Southernwood – hormonal agent, bitter digestive tonic.
- Echinacea – immune stimulant.
- Wild indigo – anti-bacterial, anti-inflammatory.
- Chamomile – relaxant, digestive tonic.

This resulted in much fewer spots, confined to outbreaks at ovulation time. Her facial hair-growth stopped increasing and energy levels improved. She hadn't had any headaches at the end of 3 months herbal medicine and continued to take this remedy for a further 3 months before stopping for a break.

Case 5 Migraines, nasal congestion and PMS

Miss H, a 30 year-old teacher, had been suffering from migraines for about four years, occurring in the week before her period or occasionally triggered by bright sunlight. Pain was central or over one eye, accompanied by nausea and a heightened sense of smell. Although regular painkillers didn't work for her, she felt slightly better in a darkened room. Miss H also noticed severe water retention in the week before her period, which was very heavy. Her feet swelled in the heat and she had to have her ears syringed frequently to relieve deafness caused by wax. She used steam inhalers to ameliorate persistent nasal congestion.

Miss H smoked 15 to 20 cigarettes daily and ate a very poor diet, consisting of scones and chocolate for breakfast, pasties for lunch and frequently missed evening meals. She drank no tea or coffee.

Discussion of her case history led us to agree that her headaches were caused by hormonal changes, venous congestion and arterial constriction, exacerbated by perennial rhinitis and smoking. She was keen to reduce her smoking habit with a view to giving up. Her diet may also have contributed to circulatory problems because it lacked vitamin C and bioflavonoids, essential nutrients for blood vessel tone and elasticity as well as helping to regulate water-balance.

The remedy

- Ground ivy – mucous membrane tonic.
- Eyebright – mucous membrane tonic.
- Feverfew – migraine reliever.
- Rue – circulatory tonic.

Miss H was also prescribed buckwheat tablets and asked to keep a dietary diary, to encourage good eating habits. This remedy brought some improvement, reducing the number and severity of headaches, but Miss H continued to smoke and her diet was still very erratic. She had bought some vitamin supplement pills and continued to take herbal medicine as well as keep a diet diary.

Case 6 Sinus headaches and insomnia

Mr R, a 43 year-old social worker, suffered continuous frontal headaches and nasal congestion, especially on one side of his face, which kept him awake at night (and his wife, who complained of his snoring!). He caught colds easily and said that he rarely finished one before the next began. The pain began when he woke in the morning and was partly relieved by a cold atmosphere or fresh air. As a result of his poor sleep he was feeling very tired, rundown and stressed. He had suffered hayfever as a teenager but it stopped when he moved from his rural home to London. He also suffered from haemorrhoids but was otherwise healthy. His diet was a little low in fruit and vegetables and rather high in meat and cheese.

We agreed that his headaches were probably due to chronic sinusitis and poor venous tone may have contributed to congestion.

The remedy

- Thyme – anti-viral, antibacterial.
- Eyebright – mucous membrane tonic.
- Elderflower – mucous membrane tonic.
- Echinacea – immune stimulant.

Mr R was also prescribed witchhazel and horsechestnut cream for piles and a steam inhalation of eucalyptus and chamomile.

This combination worked extremely well, producing total relief from symptoms in two months. Mr R returned for a repeat prescription only once, the following year after a very heavy cold.

Sources and resources

Nutrition – further reading

MAFF Manual of Nutrition (HMSO). A brief guide to the contents of major foods and dietary guidelines with daily requirements. This book was used by every home economics student and teacher from the 1950s until the 1980s when cookery and nutrition became design and labelling!

Identifying herbs – further reading

The Concise British Flora, W. Keble-Martin (Ebury Press). The author was a vicar who spent all his spare time painting wild flowers. This is a remarkable book which captures the essence of each flower and plant. Better than photos for identifying difficult to recognise subjects. Not easy to use, as the plants are arranged in families, but worth persevering.

Exercise

The British Wheel of Yoga, 25 Jermyn St, Sleaford, Lincolnshire NG34 7RU. Tel: (01529) 303233. The main association for yoga teachers and those interested in yoga. Hatha yoga is the type which has most general application – it is yoga for health. This is mainly what you will find being taught in evening classes and lunchtime sessions. It consists of a series of tone and stretch exercises which have been developed over thousands of years in India. Most teachers include some exercises from other strands of yoga as these are more directly designed to relax the mind and are associated with meditation. Some people with strong religious faiths are afraid that yoga involves taking up a mystic religion. This isn't true – the meditations are designed to make you aware of your mind and enable you to empty it. They can be performed by members of any religious group.

Seeds

King's Seeds, Monk's Farm, Coggeshall Road, Kelvedon, Essex CO5 9PG. Tel: (01376) 572456. Previously Suffolk Herbs, this is the only company in Britain selling a wide variety of wild flower and herb seeds.

Samuel Dobie and Son, Long Rd, Paignton, Devon TQ4 7SX. Tel: (01803) 696444. Dobie's Seeds sells a wide range of flower and vegetable seeds, with a good selection of culinary herbs.

Seeing herbs

The Chelsea Physic Garden, Royal Hospital Walk (entrance in Cheyne Walk), London. Tel: (0207) 352 5646. (Sloane Square tube.) Probably the best collection in Britain, begun in the seventeenth century, brilliant teas and cakes, exquisite pleasure to walk round. Open Sundays from 2pm and some weekdays. Run by volunteers (who make the cakes!).

Buying dried herbs and preparations

Alban Mills Herbs, 38 Sandridge Rd, St Albans AL1 4AS.
Tel: (01727) 858243. *www.lsgmills@care4free.net*
A very large range of medicinal and culinary herbs and
spices, creams, oils, syrups, tablets, toiletries and essential
oils. Small amounts no problem.

Gardening

The Henry Doubleday Research Association, Ryton
Gardens, Ryton in Dunsmore, near Coventry. The
Association has it's own seed catalogue, run by Chase
Organics, and a magazine for subscribers which gives
advice on organic gardening and news of organic projects
in Britain and abroad.

Gardener's Question Time, 2pm, Sunday Radio 4, repeated
in the day-time during the week, has been offering
gardening advice from a panel of experts to live audiences
for generations. *Gardener's World* is at 8.30, Friday BBC2.

Consulting herbalists

The National Institute of Medical Herbalists (NIMH) 56
Longbrook St, Exeter, Devon EX4 6AH. Tel: (01392)
426022. *www.btinternet.com/~nimh/*. Established in 1864 to
promote training and standards in herbal medicine. It is
the oldest body of professional herbalists in the world.
Members train for four years to a Bsc in Herbal Medicine,
which involves herbal pharmacology, medical sciences

and pharmacognosy (the science of recognising herbal compounds and materials).

Representatives of the NIMH sit on government committees and are involved in decisions on the safety of herbal medicines in Britain and Europe.

Counselling and talking therapies

Self-help books are abundant. You will need to read more than one to get an idea of the different sorts of talking therapies.

Patient support groups

These are extremely useful for sharing problems and solutions. Ask in your local library for the *Directory of Associations* which contains all national associations and is updated annually. The current secretarial address for the Migraine Sufferers Association is listed here.

List of herbs within their applications

Anti-migraine herbs

Feverfew

Circulatory tonics

Buckwheat
Gingko
Hawthorn
Horsechestnut
Motherwort
Rue

Rubefacient essential oils

Cedarwood
Juniper
Lavender
Pine
Rosemary
Thyme
Wintergreen

Relaxants

Chamomile
Cramp bark
Kava-kava
Lemon balm
Limeflowers
Skullcap
St John's wort
Valerian
Vervein

Digestive tonics

Chilli
Galangal
Ginger
Horseradish
Lemon balm
Rosemary
Sage
Thyme

Hormonal herbs

Anemone
Black cohosh
Chasteberry
Hops
Motherwort
Red clover
Sage
White deadnettle
Wild yam

Mucous membrane tonics

Eyebright
Elderflower
Ground ivy
Ribwort

General Index